Diabetic Diet After 50

Eating Well After 50 with Simple, Satisfying, and Sugar-Conscious Recipes to Control Type 2 Diabetes – Complete with a 45-Day Meal Plan

Clara Thompson

TABLE OF CONTENTS

Introduction

Welcome Note

Hello and welcome to "Diabetic Diet After 50"! I'm glad you're here with me as we work on improving our health together. If you've just found out you have Type 2 diabetes or want to learn how to take better care of yourself, know that you're not alone. Many people over 50 are in the same situation, and we can find ways to improve life together.

I can still recall the moment I learned I had diabetes. It felt like a storm of emotions—fear, confusion, and uncertainty—crashing in simultaneously. I had many questions: What should I make to my diet? Will my favorite meals still be available to me? With time, I learned that the key to living well with diabetes is to understand my body and make choices that help me instead of feeling restricted. This book is made for you. Inside, you'll find many helpful tips, tasty recipes, and friendly advice to help you manage your diabetes. We'll discuss the fundamental principles of healthy eating, the significance of meal planning, and how to prepare delicious meals that help manage blood sugar levels effectively. Let's begin this journey together and enjoy learning along the way!

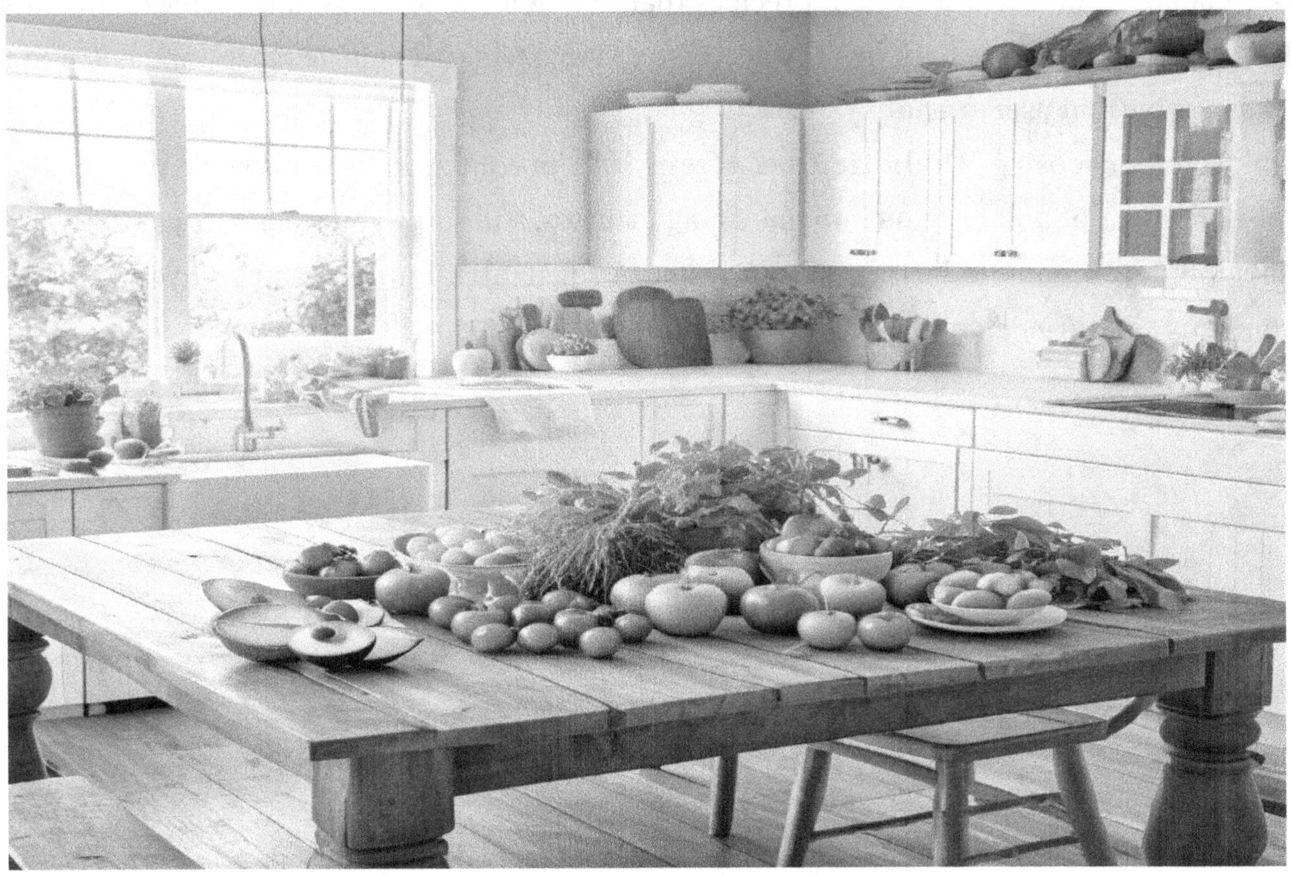

How to Use This Book

Take your time and delve into each chapter as it suits you. The book's layout is designed to be user-friendly, making it easy for you to delve into diabetes management, understand your nutritional requirements, and discover practical recipes that suit your lifestyle.

Each chapter is made for you and your unique needs as someone over 50. You'll find helpful tips for planning meals, a complete 45-day meal plan, and tasty and good recipes. When you try the recipes, look at the nutrition info, like calorie counts and options to swap ingredients to suit your taste. Feel free to make this journey your own—if some recipes look better to you, that's fine! The meal plans can be customized and interchanged to align with your tastes. Whether you're in the mood for quick snacks, filling entrees, or tasty desserts, this book is here to help you create enjoyable and health-conscious meals.

What's New in This Edition?

In this new edition of **"Diabetic Diet After 50"**, I'm excited to share many new recipes and tips about managing diabetes. You'll find recipes that focus on whole foods and balanced nutrition— delicious options that are both healthy and tasty. I've considered your feedback and ensured this book is simple and user-friendly.

Thank you for choosing **"Diabetic Diet After 50."** I'm confident that this book, with its simple meal-planning tips and insights into managing diabetes, will serve you well.

Remember, even minor adjustments can result in substantial improvements in your health. I'll accompany you throughout the journey and offer my full support!

Chapter 1: Understanding Diabetes After 50

Introduction

As we age, effectively managing Type 2 diabetes becomes more critical, particularly for individuals over 50. This chapter provides insightful and uplifting guidance on understanding the condition, its impact on aging, and the vital importance of diet in its control. Grasping and implementing these principles is crucial for safeguarding your health and overall wellbeing.

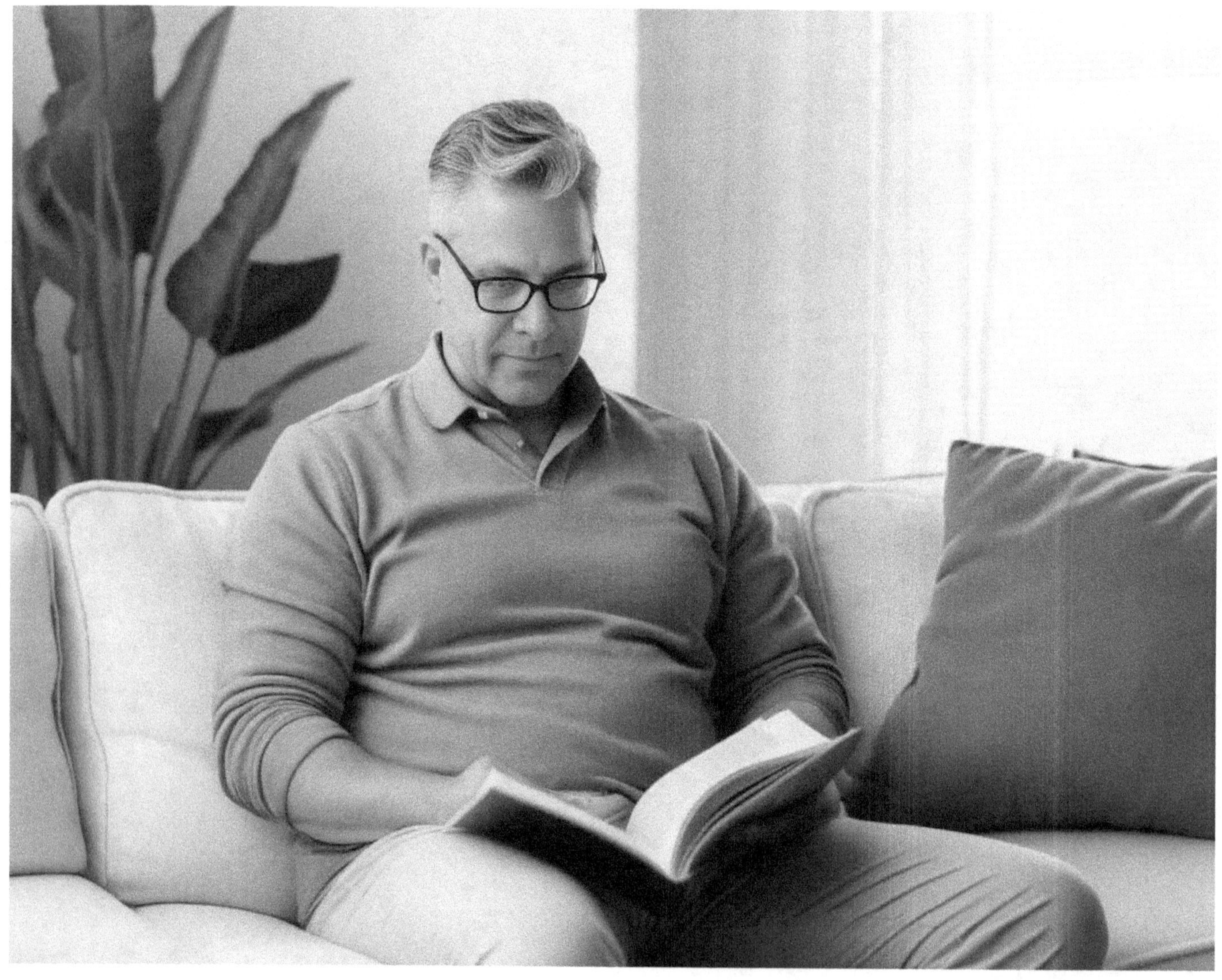

1.1 Overview of Type 2 Diabetes

Dealing with type 2 diabetes becomes increasingly complex as individuals age, particularly for those over 50. This condition, marked by insufficient insulin production or resistance to its effects, prevents glucose from entering cells effectively, essential for energy. Without proper management, glucose levels can rise dramatically, leading to serious health problems.

Unlike type 1 diabetes, which typically begins early in life due to a total lack of insulin production, type 2 diabetes often develops later in life. Lifestyle factors, including diet, physical activity, and weight, significantly influence it. This condition occurs when the body's reduced responsiveness to insulin decreases, combined with inadequate hormone production by the pancreas—a critical blood sugar regulator.

Key risk factors include being overweight, leading an inactive lifestyle, having a lineage of diabetes, and following poor eating habits. For individuals over 50, the natural slowing of metabolism and other age-related changes further increase their susceptibility to this condition. Early signs in older adults dealing with this condition, such as frequent urination, increased thirst, fatigue, unexplained weight loss, blurred vision, or slow-healing wounds, can sometimes be misinterpreted as normal aging. However, recognizing these signs is vital because ignoring them can result in more severe health issues.

In older adults, uncontrolled glucose levels can result in significant health risks, including heart disease, nerve damage, kidney issues, and vision impairment. Statistics indicate that almost one in four adults over 65 in the U.S. lives with diabetes, predominantly type 2. That underscores the importance of spreading awareness and empowering individuals to manage their health.

Adopting healthier lifestyle habits makes it possible to manage and, in some cases, even reverse type 2 diabetes. Understanding how the condition impacts your body is the first step toward making positive changes. This guide provides practical tools and insights to help you navigate life with diabetes. Remember, proactive care is the foundation for minimizing health risks and improving overall wellbeing.

1.2 How Aging Affects Diabetes

As we age, the changes in our bodies can significantly influence how we manage this type of diabetes. A slower metabolism means glucose is not processed as efficiently, requiring a more significant focus on diet and exercise to keep levels in check. The insulin response might weaken with Age, complicating blood sugar regulation. Adapting and staying proactive in addressing these changes is crucial. As metabolism slows, the body's efficiency in processing glucose diminishes. That necessitates increased mindfulness regarding diet and exercise to maintain balance. The insulin response may decline with Age, making blood sugar management more challenging. Therefore, adapting and staying proactive in managing these changes is essential. Hormonal changes with aging can also affect blood sugar regulation. Drops in hormones like estrogen and testosterone can alter insulin sensitivity and complicate weight management, underscoring the need to adapt health strategies as we age. With aging, the ability to process glucose decreases, making weight gain more accessible and maintaining consistent glucose levels more challenging. With the natural decrease in physical activity accompanying aging, making intentional adjustments to diabetes management becomes essential.

Managing this condition becomes even more critical with Age due to the increased risks of heart disease, renal issues, and nerve complications. Taking responsibility for your health is essential, as well as scheduling regular medical visits and actively participating in your care. Your doctor is a partner in managing diabetes; your involvement is vital for success. Regular visits can provide reassurance and support in your diabetes management journey. As we age, managing this form of diabetes becomes increasingly complex, especially with other conditions like hypertension and high cholesterol levels. These conditions often require different medications, which can interact and complicate treatment. Maintaining open communication with your doctor is essential for effective health management. Moreover, effective diabetes management involves more than medication; it requires lifestyle changes that improve overall health. For example, even with gentle exercises like walking, staying active can enhance insulin sensitivity and improve blood sugar regulation.

Changing eating habits and watching portion sizes can significantly impact diabetes management. It's not just about what you eat, but also how much. These minor adjustments can dramatically improve the management of this form of diabetes. While aging brings new challenges, taking charge of your wellbeing is never too late.

1.3 The Importance of Diet in Managing Diabetes

Following a well-rounded diet is crucial for effectively handling this form of diabetes. What we eat directly influences glucose levels, weight, and overall health. For individuals over 50, adopting a balanced diet is vital not only for controlling diabetes but also for preventing complications and sustaining energy levels. Understanding the role of different food groups in your diet empowers you to make choices that positively affect your health.

A well-structured diet helps maintain steady glucose levels. Focusing on carbohydrates is essential since they have the most immediate influence on blood sugar. Instead of refined carbohydrates like white bread, choose whole grains like oats, quinoa, barley, and brown rice. These complex carbohydrates digest more slowly, which helps prevent rapid fluctuations in glucose levels. Low-fat proteins like beans, fish, chicken, and tofu are crucial in stabilizing glucose levels and ensuring you feel full. Moreover, including healthy fats from avocados, nuts, olive oil, and fatty fish varieties is vital for heart health, particularly for those managing diabetes. Staying hydrated is also vital. Sometimes, feelings of hunger are a sign of dehydration. Drinking fluids consistently will prevent you from feeling hungry and overeating. You must also avoid all drinks with sugar, including soda and fruit juice, which cause a surge in your blood sugar. Instead, drink water, unsweetened tea, or lemon or cucumber water.

Healthy weight loss is another central feature of managing diabetes in older Age. Portion control plays a key role here. Eating smaller, frequent meals can help avoid large glucose swings and stabilize metabolism. Avoiding large meals high in carbohydrates and fat will also help prevent glucose spikes.

A nutritious diet involves making food choices that nourish your body and make you feel good. It can boost your energy, make blood sugar regulation easier, and reduce your chance of complications. With the proper knowledge, you can enjoy delicious, satisfying meals while keeping your diabetes under control.

Conclusion

Understanding the details of this condition is essential for individuals over 50, as it allows them to handle their health effectively, make informed decisions, and take preventive measures to maintain their overall wellbeing. This chapter has provided a wealth of information, highlighting its characteristics and the impact of aging, and it emphasizes proper nutritional care. As we age, our bodies change, requiring a new approach to diabetes management. Armed with this knowledge, you are now better informed and knowledgeable about your condition.

Remember, wise dietary choices nourish your body and enhance your wellbeing. With the proper education and guidance, you can effectively control your diabetes and lead a healthy life.

Chapter 2: Nutritional Needs After 50

Introduction

As we get older, our dietary requirements evolve. Adapting to these changes is essential to staying healthy and preventing diabetes. This chapter explains which nutrients people over 50 need, how to adjust our diet as we age, and which foods to consume more or avoid to stay healthy.

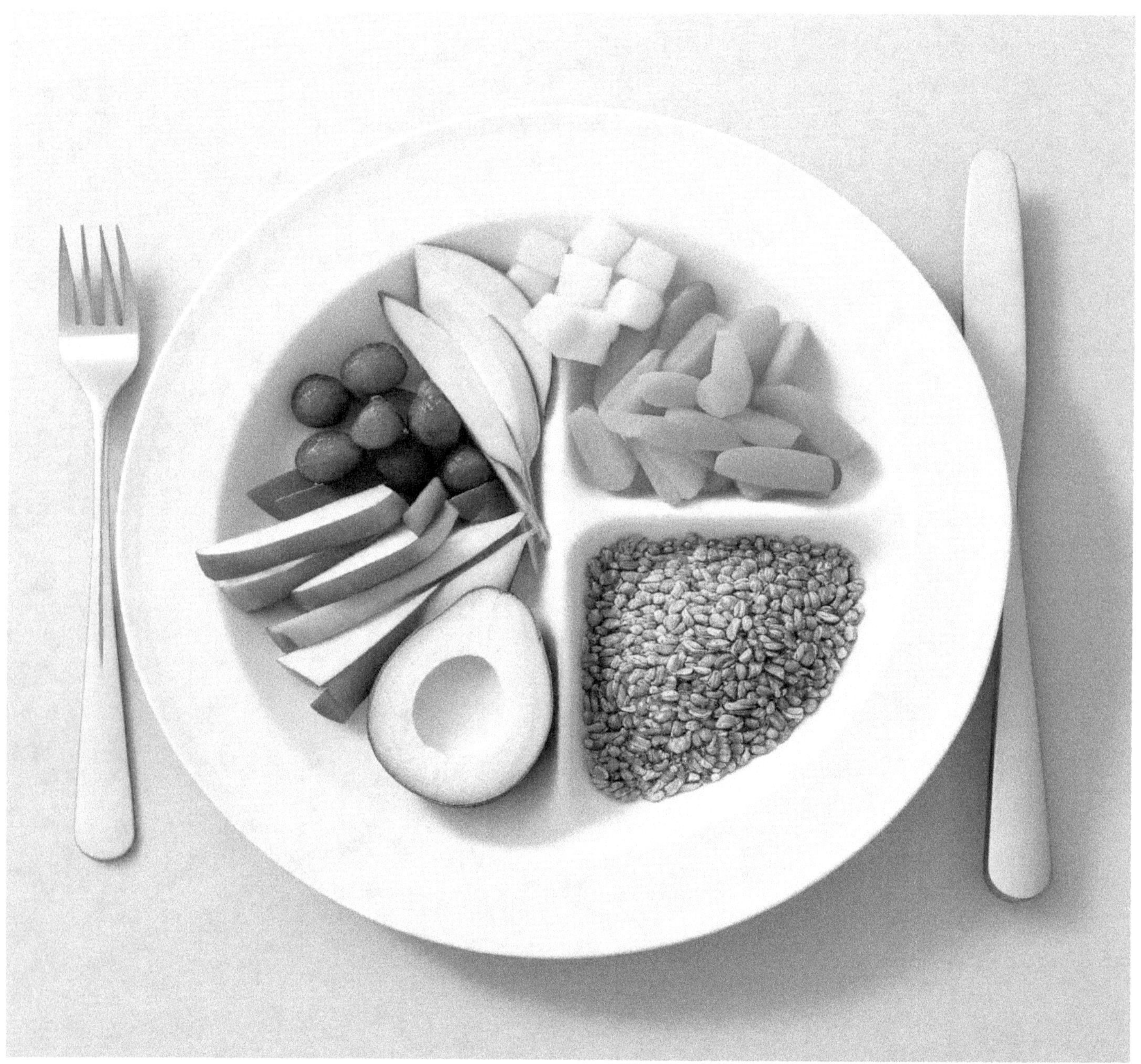

2.1 Key Nutrients and Their Roles

Understanding the essential nutrients for our health as we Age helps us make informed dietary choices. Carbs, proteins, and fats provide energy, while vitamins and minerals are necessary for health. Managing diabetes requires attention to these nutrients to maintain overall wellbeing.

Carbohydrates. Choose complex carbohydrates instead of sugary snacks and white bread. Whole grains, legumes, and vegetables are great options as they provide a more stable release of energy and are rich in fiber, which helps regulate glucose levels. Including foods like brown rice, quinoa, and whole-grain bread in your diet can offer sustained energy and keep you feeling fuller longer.

Proteins As we age, the role of protein in maintaining our muscles and strength becomes even more critical. Fish, poultry, beans, and low-fat dairy provide excellent sources of lean proteins. These proteins are beneficial as they aid in tissue repair and support the production of vital enzymes and hormones. Adding protein to meals can help control glucose levels and reduce hunger, especially for those managing diabetes. Ensuring a good amount of protein in every meal is critical to maintaining muscle health.

Healthy Fats: To maintain a healthy heart and overall fitness, you must include beneficial fats. Excellent options for these beneficial fats are nuts, avocados, and olive oil. These can alleviate inflammation and decrease the risk of cardiovascular issues, a common concern for those managing diabetes. Reducing saturated fats from beef and whole milk products, along with avoiding trans fats typically found in processed foods, can significantly improve your health and help manage diabetes more effectively.

Vitamins and Minerals. Micronutrients are crucial for sustaining health. As we age, specific vitamins and minerals become increasingly important. Vitamin D supports bone health. You can obtain Vitamin D from sunlight, fortified foods, and fatty fish. It aids in calcium absorption, ensuring your bones remain strong and healthy. Calcium supports bone density and can be sourced from dairy products and leafy greens. B vitamins, particularly B12, are essential for energy production and nerve health. Older adults should monitor their B12 levels, as absorption may decline with Age. Adding a diverse selection of fruits and vegetables to your meals is a great way to provide your body with essential nutrients.

A balanced diet with crucial macronutrients and micronutrients is necessary for individuals over fifty. Emphasizing whole, minimally processed foods supports overall health and aids in effectively managing diabetes.

2.2 Adjusting Your Diet as You Age

As we age, our nutritional needs and how we process food change due to various physiological shifts. Understanding these changes is critical to effectively adjusting our diets and maintaining good health. Adapting to these evolving nutritional needs can significantly enhance our overall wellbeing. A shift among them is slower metabolism—not burning food nearly as fast as we once did when we were young. This moderation can also lead to fat accumulation if calories aren't regulated in concert. An emphasis on nutrient-dense foods with fewer calories, such as leafy greens, beans, and low-fat dairy, is required to maintain this control. Highlight the significance of integrating entire foods into your diet. Fruits, vegetables, lean proteins, and fiber-rich grains are crucial for maintaining health and wellbeing. These options supply essential nutrients without extra calories, reassuring you about your dietary choices. They are vital in diabetes management by delivering a consistent energy supply and regulating blood sugar levels.

Taste and Appetite: Aging changes can alter our taste preferences and appetite. Many individuals find that some flavors lose their appeal, making maintaining a balanced diet more challenging. Various seasonings can enhance food flavor without adding extra calories or sodium. For instance, garlic, basil, or chili can make vegetables and lean proteins much more enjoyable.

Hydration: Our dietary requirements evolve as we age, and our bodies process food differently. Knowing about these changes is essential to fine-tuning our diet for better health. Adapting to these new dietary requirements can significantly boost our overall wellbeing. Consuming vegetables and fruits that are high in water content promotes proper hydration and provides essential nutrients that improve general wellbeing. These decisions promote general health and are especially helpful in managing diabetes. Staying hydrated is a proactive step that can make you feel responsible for your wellbeing. It's a simple yet powerful way to ensure your body functions at its best.

Portion Control: Pay attention to portion sizes, mainly as your caloric needs decrease with Age. While consuming enough nutrients is important, avoiding overeating is equally essential. Opting for smaller plates aids in managing portions, and listening to your body's hunger signals can guide you in determining the appropriate amount to eat. Eating more slowly can prevent overeating and keep you satisfied. Grasping portion control's significance empowers you, fostering a sense of responsibility for your health. Adjusting your dietary habits over time is a gradual process that requires ongoing attention.

Understanding your body's changes and making informed nutritional choices, you can stay healthy and effectively manage diabetes.

2.3 Foods to Emphasize and Foods to Avoid

Empower yourself by choosing your foods wisely, which is crucial for diabetes control and overall wellbeing. By identifying critical foods and those with negative impacts, you can establish a proper diet that promotes diabetes control and gives you control over your health.

Foods to Emphasize: Prioritizing whole grains is essential. Adding grains like quinoa, brown rice, and whole wheat can boost fiber intake. Fiber supports healthy digestion by ensuring regular bowel movements and helps regulate glucose levels by slowing down the absorption of sugar. These regulations are also crucial for health. Opt for skinless poultry, fish, legumes, and tofu as primary protein sources. These choices have less saturated fat and offer the nutrients required to maintain muscle mass. Adding a variety of vibrant foods to your meals is beneficial. These foods are not just delicious, but they also provide essential nutrients that enhance your overall health. Don't overlook beneficial fats; they're important, too. Incorporating foods like avocados, almonds, and olive oil into your meals can boost heart health and aid in managing blood. Choosing dairy products with reduced fat ensures you get the essential nutrients needed to maintain strong bones. The variety in your diet will inspire you to explore new foods and keep your meals interesting.

Foods to Avoid: Some specific foods and ingredients should be restricted or excluded to support optimal health. Limiting processed sugars is crucial to preventing blood sugar spikes. Opt for healthier alternatives to sugary drinks, desserts, and candy for better health. For instance, you can replace sugary sodas with sparkling water or unsweetened tea and swap high-sugar desserts with fresh fruits or homemade treats sweetened with natural alternatives like stevia or honey. Limiting refined carbohydrates is equally essential. Consuming white bread, pastries, and other refined grains can rapidly spike blood glucose levels while offering little nutritional value. It's critical to limit unhealthy fats, especially trans fats and large amounts of saturated fats found in fried foods and fatty meats, as these can increase the likelihood of cardiovascular disease, a significant concern for those managing diabetes. Also, monitoring sodium intake is crucial, as high sodium levels can cause high blood pressure.

Be cautious with processed foods and restaurant meals, and try to use fresh ingredients if possible to help reduce sodium.

Alcohol Consumption: A final consideration is alcohol consumption. Moderate consumption is acceptable, but the amount needs to be monitored because liquor can also change glucose levels and the response to diabetes drugs. Discussing your drinking habits with a medical professional to understand what's best for you is always a good idea. By choosing nutritious foods and eliminating foods that are harmful to health, individuals can create a healthy eating plan for managing diabetes and wellbeing.

Final Thoughts: Understanding your nutritional needs after fifty is vital and reassuring. It's the key to staying healthy and managing diabetes effectively. You can live a healthy and fulfilling life by emphasizing essential nutrients, making intelligent dietary changes, and selecting the right foods. Even minor, gradual adjustments can significantly improve your overall wellbeing, giving you a sense of security in your health journey. Gaining knowledge about nutrition boosts your confidence in making healthy choices, and embracing these changes can significantly improve your lifestyle. Whether enjoying a nutritious meal or feeling energized after physical activity, the journey to better health is enriching. Incorporating these nutritional insights into your everyday habits can help make aging a smoother and more pleasurable experience. With dedication and support, managing diabetes can become a simple process, allowing you to thrive and enjoy life to the fullest.

Chapter 3: The Role of Diet in Diabetes Control

Introduction

Effectively managing diabetes after age 50 requires a thorough understanding of how different foods impact blood sugar levels. This chapter examines the effects of carbohydrates, proteins, and fats on blood sugar, explores the Glycemic Index (GI) concept, and guides balancing meals for optimal blood sugar control. By the end, you'll know how to adjust your diet to maintain your health and successfully regulate Type 2 diabetes.

3.1 The Impact of Carbohydrates, Proteins, and Fats

When managing diabetes, it's essential to understand the function of the three main macronutrients: carbohydrates, proteins, and healthy fats. Carbohydrates often get the most attention because they directly impact glucose levels.

Carbohydrates: The Primary Source of Glucose

Carbohydrates, commonly known as carbs, are the body's primary energy source, breaking down into glucose during digestion. However, carbohydrates vary in their effects. They are classified into two categories: simple sugars and complex carbohydrates. Simple sugars in sugary snacks, soda, and processed foods are swiftly absorbed into your bloodstream, causing rapid increases in glucose levels. Unlike simple sugars, complex carbs in whole grains, veggies, and legumes metabolize more gradually, slowly releasing glucose. For individuals managing diabetes, opting for complex carbohydrates over simple ones can help avoid sudden rises in blood glucose. Choosing wholegrain bread over white bread or brown rice instead of white rice can significantly improve your health. These healthier alternatives are packed with fiber, which aids digestion and helps stabilize glucose levels.

Proteins: Supporting Satiety and Gradual Blood Sugar Changes

Proteins, another essential macronutrient, have a slower and steadier effect on glucose levels than carbohydrates. Consuming adequate protein can promote a sense of fullness for extended periods, decreasing the temptation to overeat or indulge in high-carb snacks that could affect your glucose levels. This feeling of fullness, known as 'satiety,' is crucial to managing diabetes as it can help control portion sizes and prevent sudden glucose spikes. Great options for lean protein include chicken, turkey, fish, eggs, lentils, and tofu. They keep you satisfied and have minimal effects on glucose levels.

Combined with moderate complex carbohydrates, they contribute to a balanced meal, supporting steady energy levels and glucose management.

Healthy Fats: Slowing Digestion and Enhancing Flavor

Healthy fats are essential in diabetes management because they slow digestion and help you feel satisfied after meals. While they do not directly raise glucose levels, they influence how your body metabolizes other nutrients, including carbohydrates. Incorporating beneficial fats from extra virgin olive oil, nuts, avocados, and seeds can support better glucose regulation, ensuring a more gradual energy release. It's essential to focus on unsaturated fats from sources like olive oil, fatty fish, and nuts while cutting back on trans fats and saturated fats, commonly present in processed and fried foods. Healthy fats are essential for managing glucose levels and supporting cardiovascular health, especially for those more susceptible to heart disease. By understanding how these macronutrients interact with your body, you can make more informed choices that promote stable glucose levels. Ensure your diet balances carbohydrates, proteins, and healthy fats.

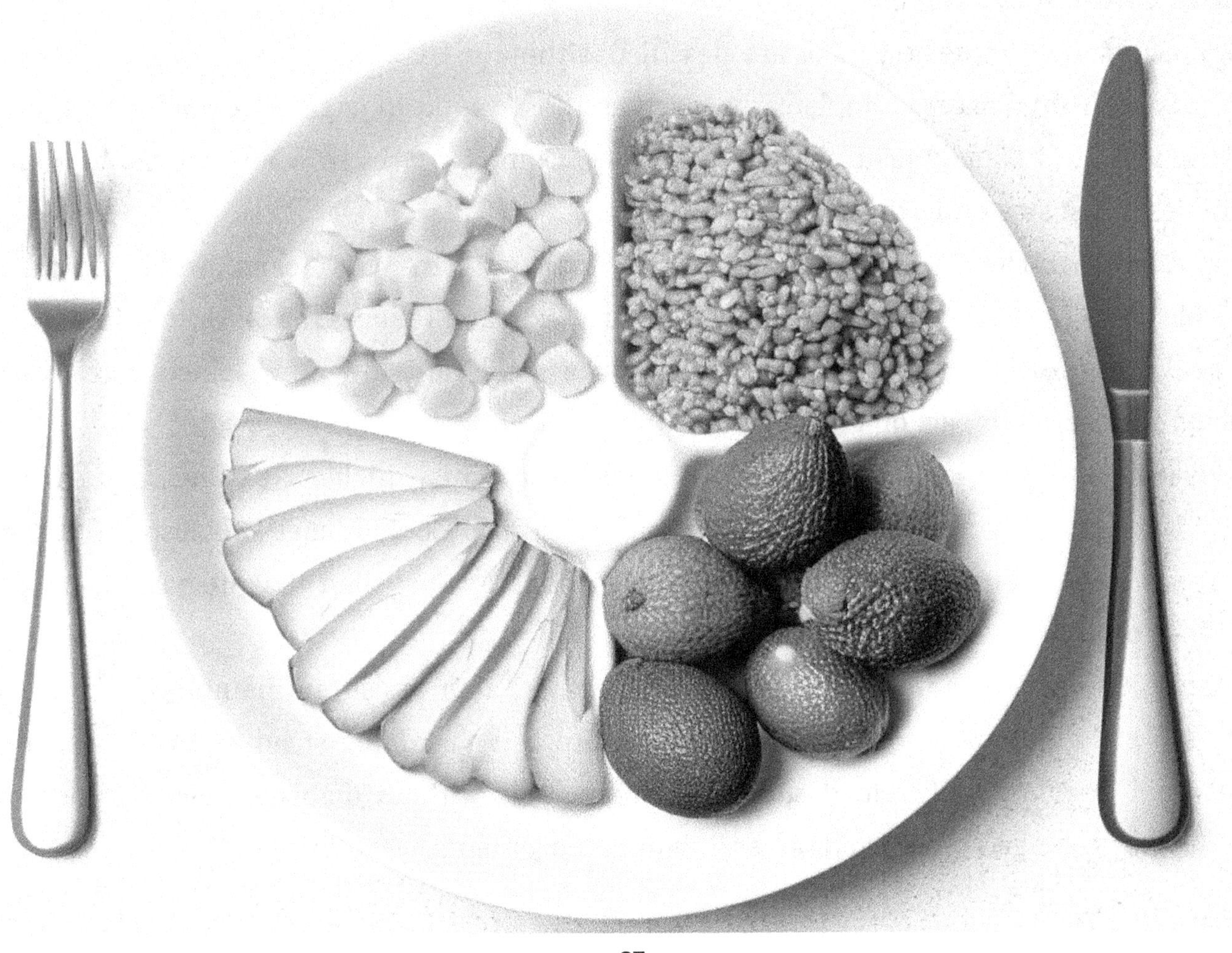

3.2 Understanding the Glycemic Index (GI)

GI is a system that evaluates how various foods influence blood glucose. It measures the speed at which carbohydrates in foods transform into glucose and enter the bloodstream. Foods that digest quickly can cause a sudden surge in blood sugar, while those that metabolize gradually release sustained energy.

How the GI Scale Works

Foods are evaluated using a range between 0 and 100, reflecting how they impact blood glucose levels. High-GI foods score above 70 and produce a rapid and notable spike in blood glucose. Low-GI foods, which score below 55, release glucose gradually, ensuring a consistent energy supply. Foods with a medium GI score fall within the range of 56-69.

For example, consuming a high-GI food like candy is akin to rapidly pouring a bucket of water into a small container, leading to an immediate overflow that represents a sharp rise in blood sugar followed by a drop. Conversely, eating an apple (a low-GI food) is like a steady water drip into the container, providing a gradual and stable energy release.

Factors Influencing the GI

Several factors determine how foods are classified within the GI:

Type of Carbohydrates: Simple carbs, such as those found in sugary treats or white bread, digest quickly and usually result in high GI values. Complex carbs in whole grains, beans, and vegetables digest slower, leading to lower GI values.

Fiber Content: Dietary fiber is essential for managing the GI. Beans, whole fruits, and vegetables are high in dietary fiber, which slows digestion and reduces the GI rating.

Fat and Protein: Including fats or proteins in a meal can slow down glucose absorption, reducing the overall impact on glucose levels.

Processing and Preparation: Processed foods often exhibit higher GI values. For instance, polished rice typically has a better GI than wholegrain rice. Cooking methods also influence GI values; pasta cooked until very soft tends to have higher GI values than al dente pasta.

The Role of GI in Health

Evaluating GI values is vital for diabetes management, as it assists in maintaining consistent glucose levels. Prioritizing foods with a low GI score and sustaining steady energy levels helps avoid rapid fluctuations in blood sugar. For individuals without diabetes, low-GI foods offer benefits like prolonged satiety and better weight management.

Conversely, consuming high-GI foods can rapidly decline energy levels, often leading to a quick appetite return. That may result in overeating or opting for less nutritious snacks. Low-GI foods include lentils, nuts, vegetables, and grains like oats and quinoa. Medium-GI foods might include bananas and rye bread, while high-GI foods typically consist of white bread, sugary cereals, and potatoes.

Balancing the GI in Meals

Combining foods with varying glycemic index levels can help create balanced meals. For example, pairing a high-GI food like polished rice with vegetables abundant in fiber and lean proteins, such as chicken, can help stabilize the overall effect on glucose levels.

Understanding and implementing GI concepts allows you to make better nutritional choices that enhance your health and vitality.

3.3 Balancing Meals for Blood Sugar Control

Maintaining consistent glucose levels is critical for managing diabetes, and balancing meals plays a significant role. Here are some guidelines to help create well-balanced meals:

Add Protein: Proteins are essential for slowing down carbohydrate digestion and avoiding sudden surges in blood glucose. Some great sources include chicken, fish, beans, tofu, and eggs. Try to have protein in every meal. For instance, top your salad with grilled chicken or pair fish with some veggies.

Choose Whole Grains: Unrefined grains digest more slowly than refined grains, stabilizing blood sugar levels. Examples include brown rice, whole wheat bread, quinoa, and oats. Incorporate whole grains regularly into your meals. For example, choose brown rice over white rice or go for whole wheat pasta instead of the regular variety.

Add Plenty of Vegetables: Veggies are abundant in vitamins, minerals, and dietary fiber. Fiber is essential as it slows the absorption of sugar into the blood. For every meal, cover at least half of your plate with vegetables. Great options include leafy greens, carrots, broccoli, and bell peppers. Incorporate different colors and kinds to get a diverse array of nutrients.

Include Healthy Fats: Fats from avocados, nuts, seeds, and olive oil help slow digestion and maintain steady glucose levels. Use them in moderation to enhance your meals. For example, add avocado slices to your sandwich or sprinkle a few nuts on your yogurt.

Watch Portion Sizes: Eating large portions can cause fluctuations in glucose levels. It's essential to be mindful of portions and stick to recommended amounts. Using smaller plates and measuring servings can help you control portions better. For instance, a serving of cooked grains is usually around half a cup, and a portion of protein should be roughly the size of your hand.

Mix Food Groups: Mixing various foods can lead to balanced meals that help keep glucose levels steady. For instance, eating a high-GI food like polished rice with fiber-packed greens and lean meats, such as chicken, can balance the overall effect on glucose levels. Similarly, including a source of healthy fats can further slow digestion and promote steady energy release.

Stay Hydrated: Drinking enough water is essential for overall well-being and can assist in regulating glucose levels. Set a target to drink at least eight glasses of water daily. Avoid sugary beverages and choose water, herbal teas, or other low-calorie drinks.

Following these guidelines and creating balanced meals can improve glucose control and well-being. Making informed decisions about your diet and how you combine different foods can dramatically impact your diabetes management and foster a healthy lifestyle.

Chapter 4: Breakfast Recipes

Introduction

For those managing diabetes, especially individuals over 50, breakfast is crucial. It kickstarts the day by providing energy and helping to stabilize blood sugar levels. A nutritious breakfast can prevent glucose spikes and crashes resulting from skipped meals or poor food choices. Additionally, as metabolism slows with age, beginning the day with a healthy, well-balanced meal can enhance overall glucose control.

This chapter offers a variety of simple, satisfying breakfast options for people over 50 managing diabetes. Each recipe is crafted to reduce unhealthy fats while ensuring excellent dietary fiber, protein sources, and beneficial fats, keeping you full and nourished. Let's explore three categories of breakfast recipes: Simple Starters, Quick & Nutritious Smoothies, and Low-Carb Hot-Breakfasts.

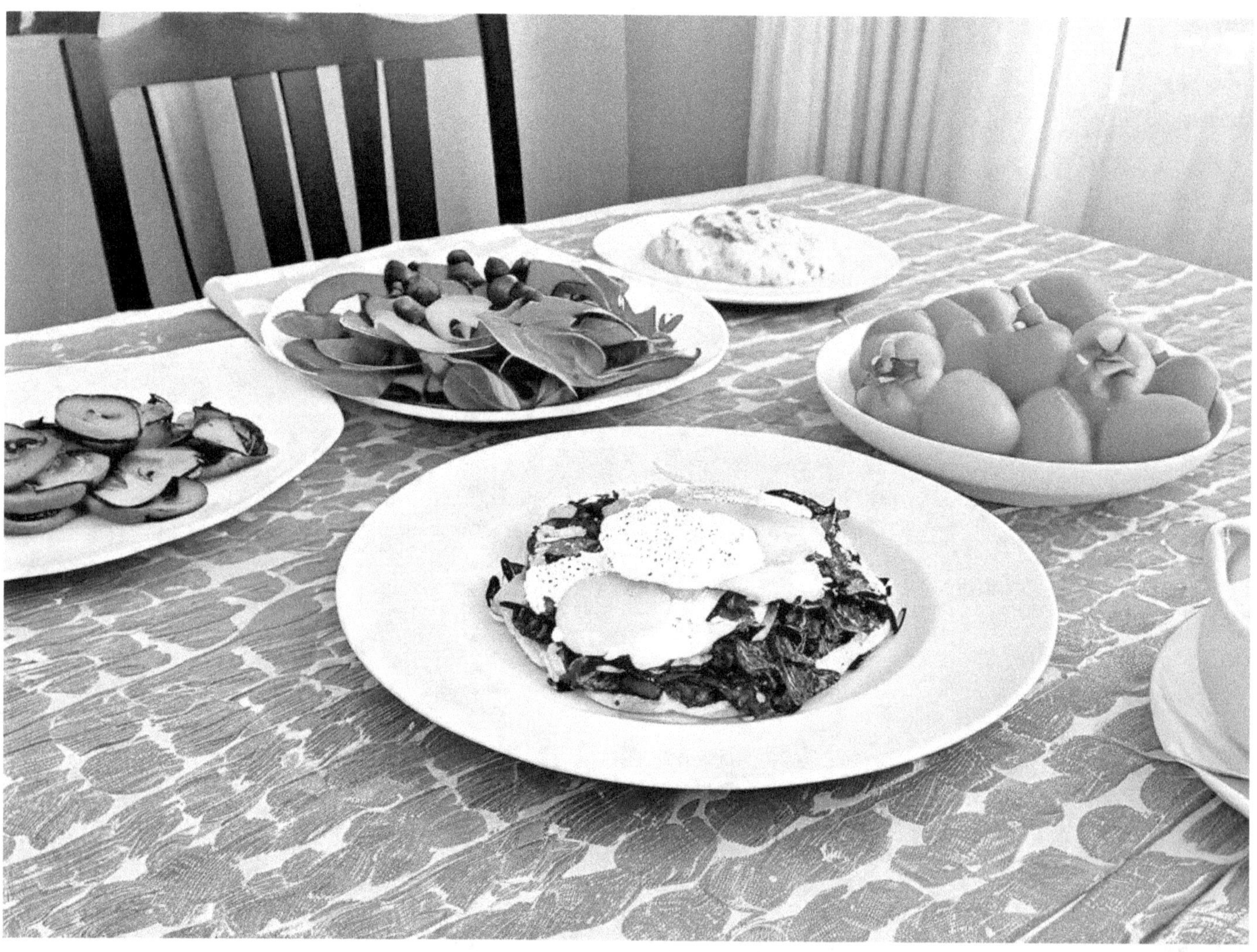

4.1: Simple Starters

These recipes are perfect for mornings when you're short on time but still need a nutritious breakfast to manage diabetes. They emphasize nutrient-dense foods, quick preparation, balanced macronutrients, and maintaining steady glucose throughout the day.

Recipe 1: Avocado and Egg Toast

Preparation Time: 10 minutes | **Servings:** 1

Ingredients: • One slice of whole grain bread • 1/2 avocado, mashed • One egg, poached or scrambled • Salt and pepper, as preferred • 1 teaspoon olive oil

Directions:

- Toast the whole grain bread.
- Season the mashed avocado with salt, then spread it onto the toast.
- Cook the egg as desired (poached or scrambled) and place it atop the avocado toast.
- Drizzle with olive oil and add pepper to taste.

Nutritional Values: • Calories: 300 • Fat: 20g (18g healthy fats, 2g unhealthy fats) • Carbohydrates: 20g • Fiber: 8g • Protein: 12g • Sugar: 2g

Recipe 2: Greek Yogurt with Flaxseeds and Berries

Preparation Time: 5 minutes | **Servings:** 1

Ingredients: • One cup of unsweetened Greek yogurt • One tablespoon of ground flaxseeds • 1/4 cup mixed berries (blueberries, raspberries) • One teaspoon of honey (optional)

Directions:

- In a bowl, combine Greek yogurt and flaxseeds.
- Add fresh mixed berries on top.
- If preferred, add a drizzle of honey.

Nutritional Values: • Calories: 250 • Fat: 10g (8g healthy fats, 2g unhealthy fats) • Carbohydrates: 22g • Fiber: 7g • Protein: 15g • Sugar: 8g

Recipe 3: Cottage Cheese and Tomato Salad

Preparation Time: 5 minutes | **Servings:** 1

Ingredients: • 1/2 cup low-fat cottage cheese • One medium-sized tomato, sliced • Fresh basil leaves • Salt and pepper for seasoning

Directions:

- Spoon cottage cheese into a bowl.
- Lay tomato slices on top.
- Garnish with fresh basil leaves, and season as desired.

Nutritional Values: • Calories: 180 • Fat: 6g (5g healthy fats, 1g unhealthy fats) • Carbohydrates: 8g • Fiber: 2g • Protein: 20g • Sugar: 5g

Recipe 4: Almond Butter and Banana Toast

Preparation Time: 5 minutes | **Servings:** 1

Ingredients: • One slice whole wheat bread• One tablespoon of almond butter • 1/2 small banana, sliced

Directions:

- Toast the bread.
- Spread almond butter on the toast, then place banana slices on top.

Nutritional Values:• Calories: 290 • Fat: 12g (10g healthy fats, 2g unhealthy fats) • Carbohydrates: 35g • Fiber: 8g • Protein: 9g • Sugar: 10g

Recipe 5: Hard-Boiled Eggs with Veggies

Preparation Time: 10 minutes | **Servings:** 1

Ingredients: • Two hard-boiled eggs • One small cucumber, sliced • 1/2 bell pepper, sliced • Salt and pepper

Directions:

- Slice the hard-boiled eggs.
- Arrange the eggs with cucumber and bell pepper slices on a plate.
- Season with a bit of salt and pepper, as preferred.

Nutritional Values:• Calories: 220 • Fat: 12g (10g healthy fats, 2g unhealthy fats) • Carbohydrates: 5g • Fiber: 2g • Protein: 16g • Sugar: 2g

4.2 Quick & Nutritious Smoothies

These easy starter recipes are ideal for mornings when you're in a rush but still need a healthy, diabetes-friendly breakfast. These recipes emphasize nutrient-dense foods, quick preparation, balanced macronutrients, and maintaining steady glucose throughout the day.

Recipe 1: Green Power Smoothie

Preparation Time: 5 minutes | **Servings:** 1

Ingredients: • 1 cup spinach • 1/2 cucumber • 1/2 avocado • 1 cup of almond milk without added sugar • One measured tablespoon of chia seeds

Directions:

- Blend all ingredients until thoroughly combined.
- Refrigerate before serving.

Nutritional Values:• Calories: 250 • Fat: 14g (12g healthy fats, 2g unhealthy fats) • Carbohydrates: 15g • Fiber: 8g • Protein: 5g • Sugar: 2g

Recipe 2: Berry and Almond Smoothie

Preparation Time: 5 minutes | **Servings:** 1

Ingredients: • 1/2 cup mixed berries (strawberries, blueberries) • 1/4 cup Greek yogurt • One tablespoon with almond butter • 1 cup of almond milk without added sugar

Directions:

- Blend all ingredients until smooth.
- Serve immediately.

Nutritional Values:• Calories: 280 • Fat: 10g (8g healthy fats, 2g unhealthy fats) • Carbohydrates: 30g • Fiber: 9g • Protein: 12g • Sugar: 10g

Recipe 3: Peanut Butter and Banana Smoothie

Preparation Time: 5 minutes | **Servings:** 1

Ingredients: • One small banana • One tablespoon of peanut butter (unsweetened) • 1/2 cup of almond milk without added sugar • One tablespoon of ground flaxseeds

Directions:

- Blend all ingredients until smooth.

- Serve chilled.

Nutritional Values: • Calories: 320 • Fat: 12g (10g healthy fats, 2g unhealthy fats) • Carbohydrates: 38g • Fiber: 10g • Protein: 10g • Sugar: 12g

Recipe 4: Tropical Smoothie

Preparation Time: 5 minute | **Servings:** 1

Ingredients: • 1/4 cup of pineapple pieces • 1/4 cup mango slices • 1/2 cup coconut water • One measured tablespoon of chia seeds

Directions:

- Blend all ingredients until smooth.
- Serve chilled.

Nutritional Values: • Calories: 200 • Fat: 8g (7g healthy fats, 1g unhealthy fats) • Carbohydrates: 30g • Fiber: 7g • Protein: 4g • Sugar: 15g

Recipe 5: Cocoa Almond Smoothie

Preparation Time: 5 minutes | **Servings:** 1

Ingredients: • One tablespoon of unsweetened cocoa powder • One tablespoon with almond butter • 1 cup of almond milk without added sugar • One measured tablespoon of chia seeds

Directions:

- Blend all ingredients until smooth.
- Serve immediately.

Nutritional Values: • Calories: 260 • Fat: 15g (13g healthy fats, 2g unhealthy fats) • Carbohydrates: 20g • Fiber: 9g • Protein: 8g • Sugar: 4g

4.3. Low-Carb Hot Breakfasts

Warm, low-carb breakfasts keep you full and your blood sugar steady. These recipes offer comfort and minimize carbs and unhealthy fats, perfect for managing diabetes without compromising taste.

Recipe 1: Veggie Omelette

Preparation Time: 10 minutes | **Servings:** 1

Ingredients: • Two standard large eggs • 1/4 cup of finely chopped spinach • 1/4 cup of diced tomatoes • One tablespoon of feta cheese • One teaspoon of olive oil

Directions:

- Beat the eggs and add a sprinkle of salt and pepper.
- Warm a skillet with olive oil. Include the spinach and tomatoes and sauté for 2 minutes.
- Transfer the whisked eggs to the prepped pan. Cook until set, then top with feta cheese.

Nutritional Values: • Calories: 220 • Fat: 16g (14g healthy fats, 2g unhealthy fats) • Carbohydrates: 5g • Fiber: 2g • Protein: 16g • Sugar: 3g

Recipe 2: Scrambled Eggs with Smoked Salmon

Preparation Time: 10 minutes | **Servings:** 1

Ingredients: • Two standard large eggs • 1 ounce of smoked salmon, chopped • One tablespoon of cream cheese • One teaspoon of olive oil

Directions:

- Whisk the eggs.
- Add olive oil to a pan, add eggs, and scramble until half set.
- Mix the smoked salmon and cream cheese, letting it cook until everything turns creamy.

Nutritional Values: • Calories: 300 • Fat: 20g (18g healthy fats, 2g unhealthy fats) • Carbohydrates: 3g • Fiber: 1g • Protein: 22g • Sugar: 1g

Recipe 3: Low-carb Pancakes with Almond Flour

Preparation Time: 15 minutes | **Servings:** 1

Ingredients: • 1/4 cup almond flour • One large egg • 1/4 teaspoon of leavening agent • 1/4 cup of unsweetened almond milk • One teaspoon of vanilla extract

Directions:

- Combine all ingredients into a smooth mixture.
- Warm up a non-stick pan and pour in small rounds of batter.
- Cook each side until golden, about 2-3 minutes per side.

Nutritional Values: • Calories: 250 • Fat: 18g (16g healthy fats, 2g unhealthy fats) • Carbohydrates: 8g • Fiber: 4g • Protein: 10g • Sugar: 2g

Recipe 4: Spinach and Mushroom Scramble

Preparation Time: 10 minutes | **Servings:** 1

Ingredients: • Two large eggs • 1/4 cup of chopped spinach • 1/4 cup of sliced mushrooms • One tablespoon of olive oil

Directions:

- Whisk the eggs.
- Sauté mushrooms in olive oil for 2 minutes.
- Add spinach and cook until tender, then add the eggs, scrambling them until they are cooked.

Nutritional Values: • Calories: 220 • Fat: 14g (12g healthy fats, 2g unhealthy fats) • Carbohydrates: 5g • Fiber: 2g • Protein: 15g • Sugar: 1g

Recipe 5: Egg Muffins with Vegetables

Preparation Time: 20 minutes | **Servings:** 3

Ingredients: • Four large eggs • 1/2 cup of chopped bell peppers • 1/2 cup of chopped zucchini • 1/4 cup of shredded cheese

Directions:

- Bring the oven to 350°F (175°C).
- Combine all the ingredients in a bowl. Pour the mixture into a greased muffin tin, then bake for 15-20 minutes.

Nutritional Values (per muffin): • Calories: 100 • Fat: 7g (5g healthy fats, 2g unhealthy fats) • Carbohydrates: 2g • Fiber: 1g • Protein: 8g • Sugar: 1g

Conclusion

Starting your morning with a nutritious, diabetes-friendly breakfast can significantly influence your blood sugar regulation and overall health, especially as you age. These recipes, from quick smoothies to hearty hot breakfasts, are crafted to maintain balanced blood glucose and deliver essential nutrients. Whether you're after a quick breakfast for busy mornings or a fancier weekend brunch, these meals will aid in sustaining a balanced diet while still being delicious and convenient.

Remember, consistency is vital when managing Type 2 diabetes. By incorporating these recipes into your routine, you'll be better equipped to manage blood glucose levels, feel more energized throughout your day, and enhance your general wellness. Try these ideas, make them your own, and enjoy the benefits of starting your mornings right. With some planning and imagination, breakfast can be an enjoyable part of managing diabetes.

Chapter 5: Light Meals & Snacks

Introduction

For those managing Type 2 diabetes, especially after 50, including light meals and snacks in your routine is critical. These nutrient-packed options help maintain steady blood sugar and provide lasting energy throughout the day. Unlike heavier meals, light dishes like salads, soups, snacks, and sandwiches are easier to digest. They can be personalized and are perfect for promoting healthy eating.

This chapter reviews several simple, delicious, and diabetes-friendly recipes incorporating protein, healthy fats, and fiber-packed carbs. These foods are designed to be quick and agile in their ability to adapt to your way of life and lifestyle. These recipes are perfect for a late-night snack or a lunch at noon. These healthy, filling choices allow you to enjoy your meals without breaking your diet.

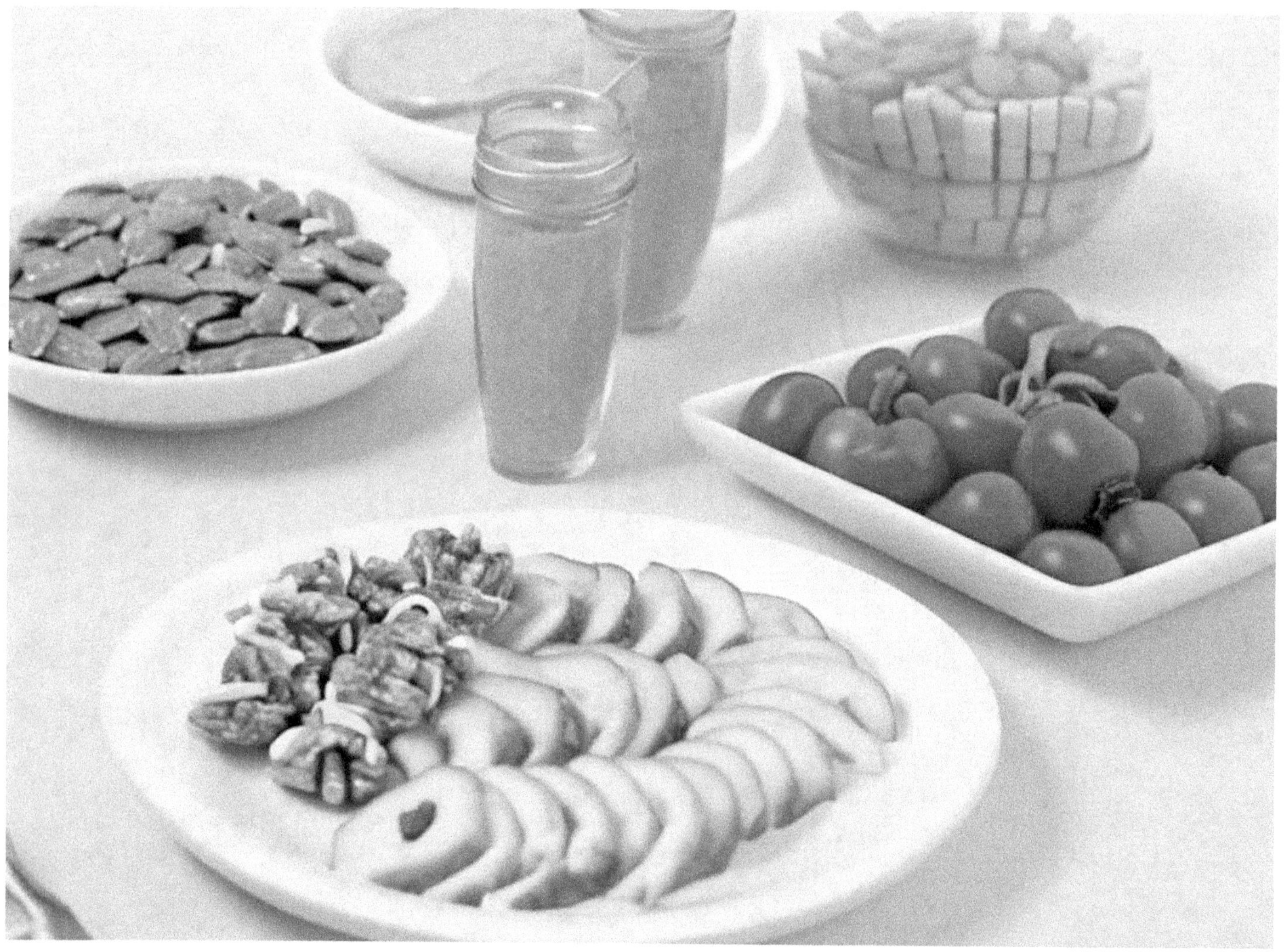

5.1: Salads and Soups

Warm, low-carb breakfasts keep you full and your blood sugar steady. These recipes offer comfort and minimize carbs and unhealthy fats, perfect for managing diabetes while still tasting great.

Recipe 1: Veggie Omelet

Preparation Time: 10 minutes | **Servings:** 1

Ingredients: • Two giant eggs • 1/4 cup of fresh diced spinach • 1/4 cup of diced tomatoes • One tablespoon of feta cheese • One teaspoon of olive oil

Directions:

- Mix the eggs and add a bit of salt and pepper.
- Warm the olive oil in a pan. Add the spinach and tomatoes and sauté for 2 minutes.
- Pour the mixed eggs into the ready pan. Cook until set, then top with feta cheese.

Nutritional Values: • Calories: 220 • Fat: 16g (14g healthy fats, 2g unhealthy fats) • Carbohydrates: 5g • Fiber: 2g • Protein: 16g • Sugar: 3g

Recipe 2: Scrambled Eggs with Smoked Salmon

Preparation Time: 10 minutes | **Servings:** 1

Ingredients: • Two giant eggs • 1 ounce of smoked salmon, chopped • One tablespoon of cream cheese • One teaspoon of olive oil

Directions:

- Whisk the eggs.
- Add olive oil to a pan, add eggs, and scramble until half set.
- Mix in the smoked salmon and cream cheese, cooking until everything becomes creamy.

Nutritional Values: • Calories: 300 • Fat: 20g (18g healthy fats, 2g unhealthy fats) • Carbohydrates: 3g • Fiber: 1g • Protein: 22g • Sugar: 1g

Recipe 3: Low-carb Pancakes with Almond Flour

Preparation Time: 15 minutes | **Servings:** 1

Ingredients: • 1/4 cup almond flour • One large egg • 1/4 teaspoon of leavening agent • 1/4 cup of unsweetened almond milk • One teaspoon of vanilla extract

Directions:

- Combine all ingredients into a smooth batter.
- Warm up a non-stick skillet and pour small rounds of batter.
- Cook each side until golden, about 2-3 minutes per side.

Nutritional Values: • Calories: 250 • Fat: 18g (16g healthy fats, 2g unhealthy fats) • Carbohydrates: 8g • Fiber: 4g • Protein: 10g • Sugar: 2g

Recipe 4: Spinach and Mushroom Scramble

Preparation Time: 10 minutes | **Servings:** 1

Ingredients: • Two giant eggs • 1/4 cup of diced spinach • 1/4 cup of sliced mushrooms • One tablespoon of olive oil

Directions:

- Whisk the eggs.
- Sauté mushrooms in olive oil for 2 minutes.
- Add spinach and sauté until wilted, then add the eggs, scrambling them until they are cooked.

Nutritional Values: • Calories: 220 • Fat: 14g (12g healthy fats, 2g unhealthy fats) • Carbohydrates: 5g • Fiber: 2g • Protein: 15g • Sugar: 1g

Recipe 5: Egg Muffins with Vegetables

Preparation Time: 20 minutes | **Servings:** 3

Ingredients: • Four large eggs • 1/2 cup of chopped bell peppers • 1/2 cup of chopped zucchini • 1/4 cup of shredded cheese

Directions:

- Set the oven to 350°F (175°C) and let it preheat.
- Combine all ingredients in a bowl. Pour the mixture into a greased muffin tin, then bake for 15-20 minutes.

Nutritional Values (per muffin): • Calories: 100 • Fat: 7g (5g healthy fats, 2g unhealthy fats) • Carbohydrates: 2g • Fiber: 1g • Protein: 8g • Sugar: 1g

5.2: Snacks and Small Bites

Healthy snacks bridge the gap between meals, keeping blood sugar levels steady all day. The following snacks are quick to prepare, nutrient-dense, and diabetic-friendly, perfect whenever you need a light bite to keep your energy up.

Recipe 1: Cucumber and Hummus Bites

Preparation Time: 5 minutes | **Servings:** 1

Ingredients: • 1/2 cucumber, sliced • Two tablespoons hummus

Directions:

- Spread hummus on cucumber slices.
- Enjoy as a refreshing, light snack.

Nutritional Values: • Calories: 100 • Fat: 5g (4g healthy fats, 1g unhealthy fats) • Carbohydrates: 12g • Fiber: 4g • Protein: 3g • Sugar: 2g

Recipe 2: Hard-boiled Egg with Veggies

Preparation Time: 10 minutes | **Servings:** 1

Ingredients: • One hard-boiled egg • 1/2 bell pepper, sliced • A hint of salt and pepper

Directions:

- Slice the egg and serve with bell pepper slices.
- Sprinkle some salt and pepper to taste.

Nutritional Values: • Calories: 120 • Fat: 8g (7g healthy fats, 1g unhealthy fats) • Carbohydrates: 5g • Fiber: 2g • Protein: 10g • Sugar: 3g

Recipe 3: Almonds and Berries

Preparation Time: 2 minutes | **Servings:** 1

Ingredients: • Ten almonds • 1/4 cup mixed berries

Directions:

- Mix almonds and berries in a compact container.
- Enjoy as a sweet and crunchy snack.

Nutritional Values: • Calories: 150 • Fat: 9g (8g healthy fats, 1g unhealthy fats) • Carbohydrates: 14g • Fiber: 6g • Protein: 5g • Sugar: 8g

Recipe 4: Celery Sticks with Peanut Butter

Preparation Time: 5 minutes | **Servings:** 1

Ingredients: • Two celery sticks • One tablespoon peanut butter (unsweetened)

Directions:

- Spread peanut butter onto celery sticks.
- Serve immediately.

Nutritional Values: • Calories: 120 • Fat: 9g (8g healthy fats, 1g unhealthy fats) • Carbohydrates: 7g • Fiber: 4g • Protein: 4g • Sugar: 2g

Recipe 5: Greek Yogurt with Walnuts

Preparation Time: 5 minutes | **Servings:** 1

Ingredients: • Half a cup of unflavored Greek yogurt • One tablespoon of walnuts, chopped

Directions:

- Stir the walnuts into the Greek yogurt.
- Enjoy as a creamy, protein-packed snack.

Nutritional Values: • Calories: 180 • Fat: 9g (8g healthy fats, 1g unhealthy fats) • Carbohydrates: 8g • Fiber: 2g • Protein: 15g • Sugar: 4g

5.3: Sandwiches and Wraps

Healthy snacks fill the gaps between meals, keeping blood sugar levels stable during the day. These snacks are quick to prepare, nutrient-dense, and diabetic-friendly, perfect whenever you need a light bite to keep your energy up.

Recipe 1: Cucumber and Hummus Bites

Preparation Time: 5 minutes | **Servings:** 1

Ingredients: • 1/2 cucumber, sliced • Two tablespoons hummus

Directions:

- Spread hummus on cucumber slices.
- Enjoy as a refreshing, light snack.

Nutritional Values: • Calories: 100 • Fat: 5g (4g healthy fats, 1g unhealthy fats) • Carbohydrates: 12g • Fiber: 4g • Protein: 3g • Sugar: 2g

Preparation Time: 10 minutes | **Servings:** 1

Ingredients: • One hard-boiled egg • 1/2 bell pepper, sliced • A hint of salt and pepper

Directions:

- Slice the egg and serve with bell pepper slices.
- Add a pinch of salt and pepper.

Nutritional Values: • Calories: 120 • Fat: 8g (7g healthy fats, 1g unhealthy fats) • Carbohydrates: 5g • Fiber: 2g • Protein: 10g • Sugar: 3g

Recipe 3: Almonds and Berries

Preparation Time: 2 minutes | **Servings:** 1

Ingredients: • Ten almonds • 1/4 cup mixed berries

Directions:

- Combine almonds and berries in a compact bowl.
- Enjoy as a sweet and crunchy snack.

Nutritional Values: • Calories: 150 • Fat: 9g (8g healthy fats, 1g unhealthy fats) • Carbohydrates: 14g • Fiber: 6g • Protein: 5g • Sugar: 8g

Recipe 4: Celery Sticks with Peanut Butter

Preparation Time: 5 minutes | **Servings:** 1

Ingredients: • Two celery sticks • One tablespoon peanut butter (unsweetened)

Directions:

- Spread peanut butter onto celery sticks.
- Serve immediately.

Nutritional Values: • Calories: 120 • Fat: 9g (8g healthy fats, 1g unhealthy fats) • Carbohydrates: 7g • Fiber: 4g • Protein: 4g • Sugar: 2g

Recipe 5: Greek Yogurt with Walnuts

Preparation Time: 5 minutes | **Servings:** 1

Ingredients: • Half a cup of plain Greek yogurt • One tablespoon of walnuts, chopped

Directions:

- Stir the walnuts into the Greek yogurt.
- Enjoy as a creamy, protein-packed snack.

Nutritional Values: • Calories: 180 • Fat: 9g (8g healthy fats, 1g unhealthy fats) • Carbohydrates: 8g • Fiber: 2g • Protein: 15g • Sugar: 4g

Conclusion

Adding light meals and snacks to your eating plan is a practical way to control blood sugar levels while ensuring you get essential nutrients throughout the day. The recipes in this chapter are designed to be simple, quick, and adaptable, making integrating them into your everyday routine effortless. Whether you're searching for a filling salad, a satisfying snack, or a convenient sandwich, these options are perfect for anyone managing Type 2 diabetes. As you explore these recipes, remember that variety is vital. Feel free to experiment with different flavors and ingredients to suit your preferences while keeping your meals balanced and nutritious. Light meals and snacks don't have to be boring; they can be flavorful, exciting, and deeply satisfying. The path to better health is made up of small, consistent steps, and by making mindful food choices, you can enjoy your meals while keeping your diabetes in check.

Chapter 6: Main Dishes

Introduction

Main dishes form the heart of a diabetes-friendly diet, especially for individuals over 50 who need nutritious and satisfying meals. These meals help maintain blood sugar levels while delivering nutrients like fiber, healthy fats, and lean proteins. Managing diabetes doesn't mean compromising on flavor or enjoyment in your meals. There are countless ways to craft delicious and health-conscious main dishes. In this chapter, you'll find various recipes that cater to different preferences, from plant-based options to protein-packed seafood, poultry, and meat dishes. Each recipe is crafted to be easy to make, delicious, and perfectly balanced for managing diabetes. With these main dishes, you can enjoy diverse ingredients and seasonings that satisfy your palate while controlling your blood sugar. Whether you're a fan of vegetarian meals, enjoy seafood, or prefer lean poultry and meat, the following recipes will inspire you to create meals that support your health and bring joy to your table. Let's explore these diabetes-friendly options together and discover how delicious eating well can be.

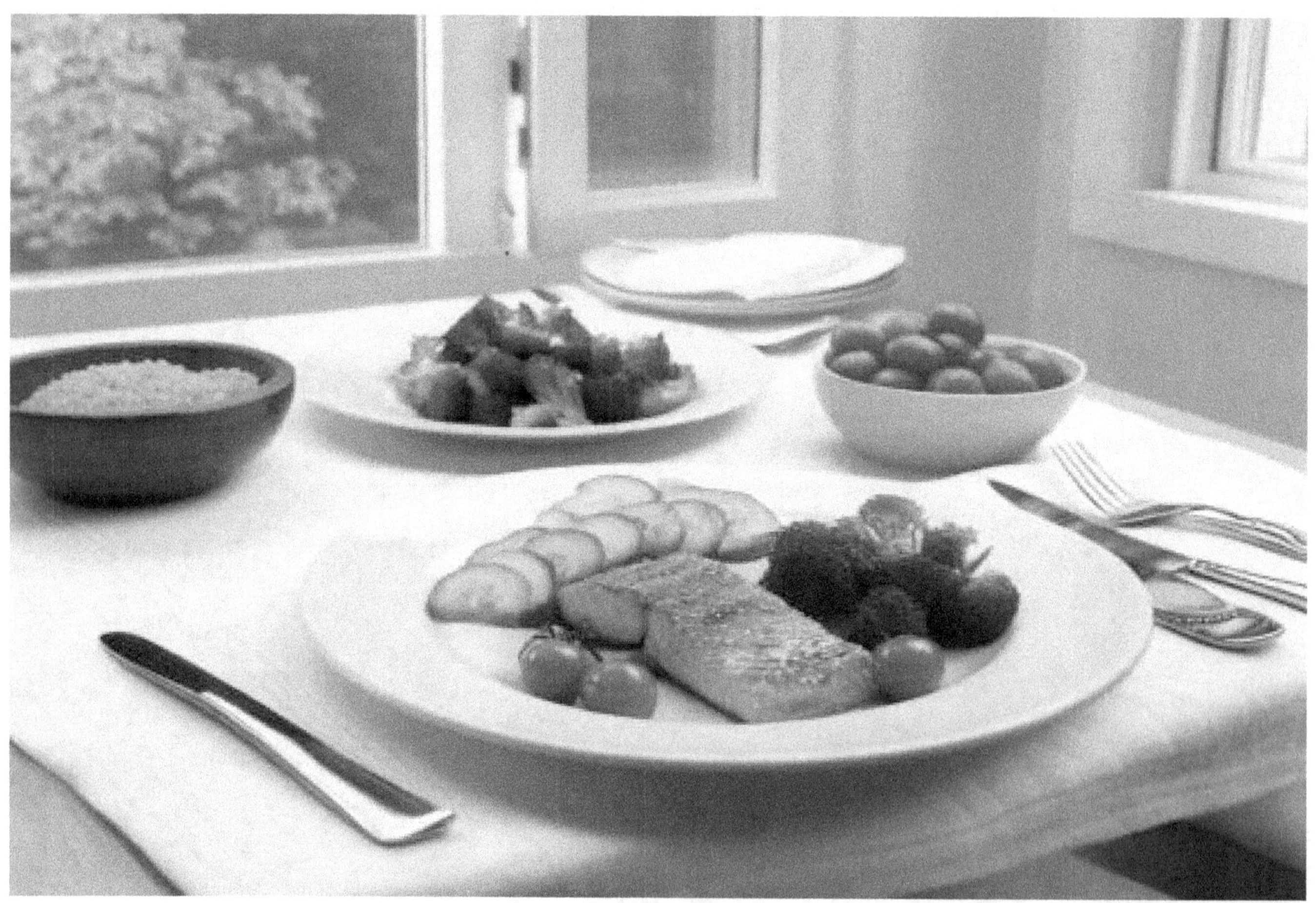

6.1: Vegetarian Delights

Plant-based meals are an excellent method to boost fiber and essential nutrient intake while maintaining a light and diabetes-friendly diet. These vegetarian main dishes are both flavorful and satisfying, perfect for those looking to add more vegetables and plant-based proteins to their meals without compromising on flavor.

Recipe 1: Lentil and Spinach Stew

Preparation Time: 25 minutes | **Servings:** 1

Ingredients: • 1/2 cup cooked lentils • 1 cup fresh spinach • 1/4 onion, chopped • One garlic clove, minced • One spoonful of olive oil • 1/2 cup vegetable stock • Salt and pepper.

Directions:

- Warm a pan with olive oil, then cook the onion and garlic until tender.
- Incorporate the lentils and vegetable stock, letting it cook on low heat for ten minutes.
- Stir in spinach and cook until wilted.
- Lightly season with salt and pepper, then serve warm.

Nutritional Values: • Calories: 280 • Fat: 8g (7g healthy fats, 1g unhealthy fats) • Carbohydrates: 40g • Fiber: 15g • Protein: 15g • Sugar: 3g

Recipe 2: Grilled Vegetable Quinoa Bowl

Preparation Time: 20 minutes | **Servings:** 1

Ingredients: • 1/4 cup quinoa • 1/2 zucchini, sliced • Half red bell pepper, sliced into thin strips • One spoonful of olive oil • One teaspoon of balsamic vinegar • Salt and pepper as needed

Directions:

- Cook the quinoa following the package instructions.
- Mix the vegetables in olive oil, then grill until they are tender.
- Mix the quinoa with the grilled vegetables, lightly drizzle with balsamic vinegar, then season to taste.

Nutritional Values: • Calories: 290 • Fat: 10g (9g healthy fats, 1g unhealthy fats) • Carbohydrates: 40g • Fiber: 8g • Protein: 9g • Sugar: 6g

Recipe 3: Stuffed Bell Peppers with Black Beans

Preparation Time: 30 minutes | **Servings:** 1

Ingredients: • One bell pepper halved • 1/4 cup of cooked black beans • 1/4 cup brown rice, cooked • One tablespoon salsa • One spoonful of olive oil • One tablespoon shredded cheese (optional)

Directions:

- Bring the oven up to 350°F (175°C).
- Mix the beans, rice, and salsa.
- Fill each half of the bell pepper with the prepared mixture.
- Coat with olive oil and roast for 20 minutes.
- Add cheese on top if desired, then serve.

Nutritional Values: • Calories: 320 • Fat: 10g (8g healthy fats, 2g unhealthy fats) • Carbohydrates: 48g • Fiber: 12g • Protein: 10g • Sugar: 5g

Recipe 4: Chickpea and Tomato Curry

Preparation Time: 25 minutes | **Servings:** 1

Ingredients: • 1/2 cup chickpeas, cooked • 1/2 cup diced tomatoes • 1/4 onion, chopped • One garlic clove, minced • One teaspoon of curry powder • 1/2 cup light coconut milk • Salt and pepper

Directions:

- Sauté the onion and garlic in a pan until softened.
- Add the chickpeas, tomatoes, and curry powder.
- Combine the coconut milk and let it gently simmer for 10 minutes.
- Season to your liking before serving.

Nutritional Values: • Calories: 300 • Fat: 12g (10g healthy fats, 2g unhealthy fats) • Carbohydrates: 35g • Fiber: 10g • Protein: 10g • Sugar: 6g

Recipe 5: Roasted Cauliflower with Tahini Sauce

Preparation Time: 25 minutes | **Servings:** 1

Ingredients: • 1/2 head cauliflower, chopped • One spoonful of olive oil • One tablespoon • tahini • One teaspoon of lemon juice • Salt and pepper

Directions:

- Bring the oven up to 350°F (175°C).
- Toss the cauliflower in olive oil, then season it to taste.
- Roast for 20 minutes until golden.
- Blend the tahini with lemon juice, then drizzle over the roasted cauliflower.

Nutritional Values: • Calories: 250 • Fat: 14g (12g healthy fats, 2g unhealthy fats) • Carbohydrates: 20g • Fiber: 8g • Protein: 6g • Sugar: 4g

6.2: Fish and Seafood

Fish and seafood provide lean protein and heart-healthy omega-3 fats, making them excellent choices for individuals with Type 2 diabetes. These recipes are light, flavorful, and packed with nutrients to support heart health and maintain balanced blood sugar levels.

Recipe 1: Grilled Salmon with Lemon

Preparation Time: 15 minutes | **Servings:** 1

Ingredients: • One salmon fillet (4 oz) • One spoonful of olive oil • One spoonful of citrus juice• Seasoning

Directions:
- Preheat the grill or a pan to medium heat.
- Brush the salmon with the mixture of oil and citrus juice.
- Season, then grill for 5-7 minutes per side.

Nutritional Values: • Calories: 280 • Fat: 16g (14g healthy fats, 2g unhealthy fats) • Carbohydrates: 1g • Fiber: 0g • Protein: 30g • Sugar: 0g

Recipe 2: Shrimp Stir-Fry with Vegetables

Preparation Time: 20 minutes | **Servings:** 1

Ingredients: • 1/2 cup shrimp, cleaned • 1/4 cup of red bell peppers, cut into thin strips • ¼ cup broccoli florets • One tablespoon of low-sodium soy sauce • One teaspoon of oil

Directions:
- Warm the oil in a pan.
- Stir-fry the shrimp for 3-4 minutes until pink.
- Add the vegetables and soy sauce, cooking for an additional 5 minutes.

Nutritional Values: • Calories: 220 • Fat: 8g (7g healthy fats, 1g unhealthy fats) • Carbohydrates: 10g • Fiber: 4g • Protein: 25g • Sugar: 3g

Recipe 3: Baked Cod with Herbs

Preparation Time: 20 minutes | **Servings:** 1

Ingredients: • One cod fillet (4 oz) • One spoonful of oil • One teaspoon of dried oregano • One spoonful of citrus juice • Seasoning

Directions:

- Set the oven to 350°F (175°C) and allow it to preheat.
- Place the cod in an ovenproof dish, pour oil over it, and add a hint of citrus juice.
- Sprinkle with oregano and seasoning, then bake for 15 minutes.

Nutritional Values: • Calories: 230 • Fat: 10g (9g healthy fats, 1g unhealthy fats) • Carbohydrates: 2g • Fiber: 0g • Protein: 30g • Sugar: 0g

Recipe 4: Tuna Salad with Avocado

Preparation Time: 10 minutes | **Servings:** 1

Ingredients: • 1/4 cup canned tuna (in water, drained) • 1/4 avocado, mashed • One spoonful of citrus juice • Seasoning

Directions:

- Combine the tuna, avocado, and citrus juice.
- Adjust the seasoning to taste.
- Serve on a bed of greens or with whole-grain crackers.

Nutritional Values: • Calories: 250 • Fat: 15g (13g healthy fats, 2g unhealthy fats) • Carbohydrates: 8g • Fiber: 6g • Protein: 22g • Sugar: 0g

Recipe 5: Seared Scallops with Asparagus

Preparation Time: 15 minutes | **Servings:** 1

Ingredients: • Five scallops • 1/4 bunch asparagus • One spoonful of oil • Seasoning

Directions:

- Warm the oil in a skillet set to medium heat.
- Sear the scallops for 2-3 minutes on each side.
- Sauté the asparagus in the same pan for 5 minutes, season, and serve together.

Nutritional Values: • Calories: 260 • Fat: 12g (10g healthy fats, 2g unhealthy fats) • Carbohydrates: 12g • Fiber: 6g • Protein: 20g • Sugar: 2g

6.3: Poultry and Meat Recipes

Poultry and lean meat are versatile options that can be prepared to support diabetes management. These recipes emphasize lean cuts and healthy cooking techniques to satisfy meals and support health goals.

Recipe 1: Grilled Chicken Breast with Herbs

Preparation Time: 20 minutes | **Servings:** 1

Ingredients: • One chicken fillet (4 oz) • One tablespoon of olive oil • One teaspoon of dried herbs (rosemary, thyme, or oregano) • Seasoning

Directions:

- Add olive oil and fresh herbs to the poultry fillet.
- Grill both sides over medium heat for 6-8 minutes.
- Season, then serve.

Nutritional Values: • Calories: 270 • Fat: 12g (10g healthy fats, 2g unhealthy fats) • Carbohydrates: 2g • Fiber: 0g • Protein: 36g • Sugar: 0g

Recipe 2: Turkey Meatballs with Tomato Sauce

Preparation Time: 30 minutes | **Servings:** 1

Ingredients: • 1/4 lb ground turkey • 1/4 cup diced onion • One garlic clove, minced • 1/2 cup tomato sauce (low-sodium) • One tablespoon of olive oil

Directions:

- Fry the meatballs in heated olive oil until golden.
- Pour tomato sauce over and simmer for 10 minutes.

Nutritional Values: • Calories: 280 • Fat: 14g (12g healthy fats, 2g unhealthy fats) • Carbohydrates: 10g • Fiber: 3g • Protein: 25g • Sugar: 4g

Recipe 3: Baked Chicken Thigh with Lemon

Preparation Time: 30 minutes | **Servings:** 1

Ingredients: • One chicken thigh, skinless • One spoonful of olive oil • One spoonful of lemon juice • Seasoning

Directions:

- Bring the oven up to 350°F (175°C).
- Coat the chicken with olive oil and lemon juice.
- Bake for 25-30 minutes until fully cooked.

Nutritional Values: • Calories: 290 • Fat: 15g (12g healthy fats, 3g unhealthy fats) Carbohydrates: 2g • Fiber: 0g • Protein: 30g • Sugar: 0g

Recipe 4: Beef Stir-Fry with Broccoli

Preparation Time: 20 minutes | **Servings:** 1

Ingredients: • 1/4 lb lean beef, thinly sliced • 1/4 cup broccoli florets • One tablespoon of soy sauce (low sodium) • One teaspoon of olive oil

Directions:

- Heat olive oil in a skillet.
- Stir-fry the beef for 3-4 minutes until browned.
- Add broccoli and soy sauce, then cook for five more minutes.

Nutritional Values: • Calories: 290 • Fat: 10g (8g healthy fats, 2g unhealthy fats) • Carbohydrates: 10g • Fiber: 4g • Protein: 30g • Sugar: 2g

Recipe 5: Pork Tenderloin with Garlic and Herbs

Preparation Time: 25 minutes | **Servings:** 1

Ingredients: • One pork tenderloin (4 oz) • One garlic clove, minced • One teaspoon of olive oil • One teaspoon of dried herbs (thyme, rosemary)

Directions:

- Rub the pork with olive oil, garlic, and herbs.
- Sauté in a skillet on medium heat for about 8 to 10 minutes, flipping often to achieve a golden-brown crust.
- Let rest for 5 minutes before slicing.

Nutritional Values: • Calories: 280 • Fat: 12g (10g healthy fats, 2g unhealthy fats) • Carbohydrates: 2g • Fiber: 0g • Protein: 36g • Sugar: 0g

Conclusion

Main dishes are the heart of every meal. For those managing Type 2 diabetes, creating nourishing and balanced dishes is crucial. The recipes in this chapter are designed to be delicious, easy to prepare, and mindful of your health needs. They allow you to savor different flavors while maintaining steady blood sugar levels.

You can explore diverse flavors and textures that make meal planning exciting and enjoyable by incorporating various ingredients—from plant-based options to lean proteins and fish. Remember that eating well with diabetes isn't restrictive; it can be an opportunity to experiment with new recipes and discover what suits your taste and lifestyle best.

We hope these main dish recipes inspire you to take control of your diet while still enjoying every bite. Keeping up a healthy, balanced diet is essential to managing diabetes effectively.

With these flavorful dishes, you can feel confident that you're nourishing your body in the best way possible.

Chapter 7: Side Dishes

Introduction

Side dishes ensure a balanced and fulfilling meal, especially for those managing Type 2 diabetes. Often overlooked, side dishes can provide essential nutrients that help stabilize blood sugar and enhance the taste and texture of the main dish. A suitable side dish can enhance any meal by providing essential vitamins, minerals, and fiber, whether nutrient-dense vegetables, fiber-rich whole grains, or legumes. This chapter highlights simple and tasty side dishes suitable for people with diabetes. Integrating these sides into your meals delivers diverse flavors and textures, all while supporting a healthy eating plan. Whether you pair them with fish, chicken, or vegetarian main courses, these side dishes are designed to enhance any meal while helping to manage your blood sugar levels. We invite you to try these recipes and ingredients to craft side dishes that match your preferences. These adaptable sides are nutritious and delicious, offering a pleasing method to uphold a balanced diet. Let's explore how to incorporate tasty and healthy side dishes into your meal plan.

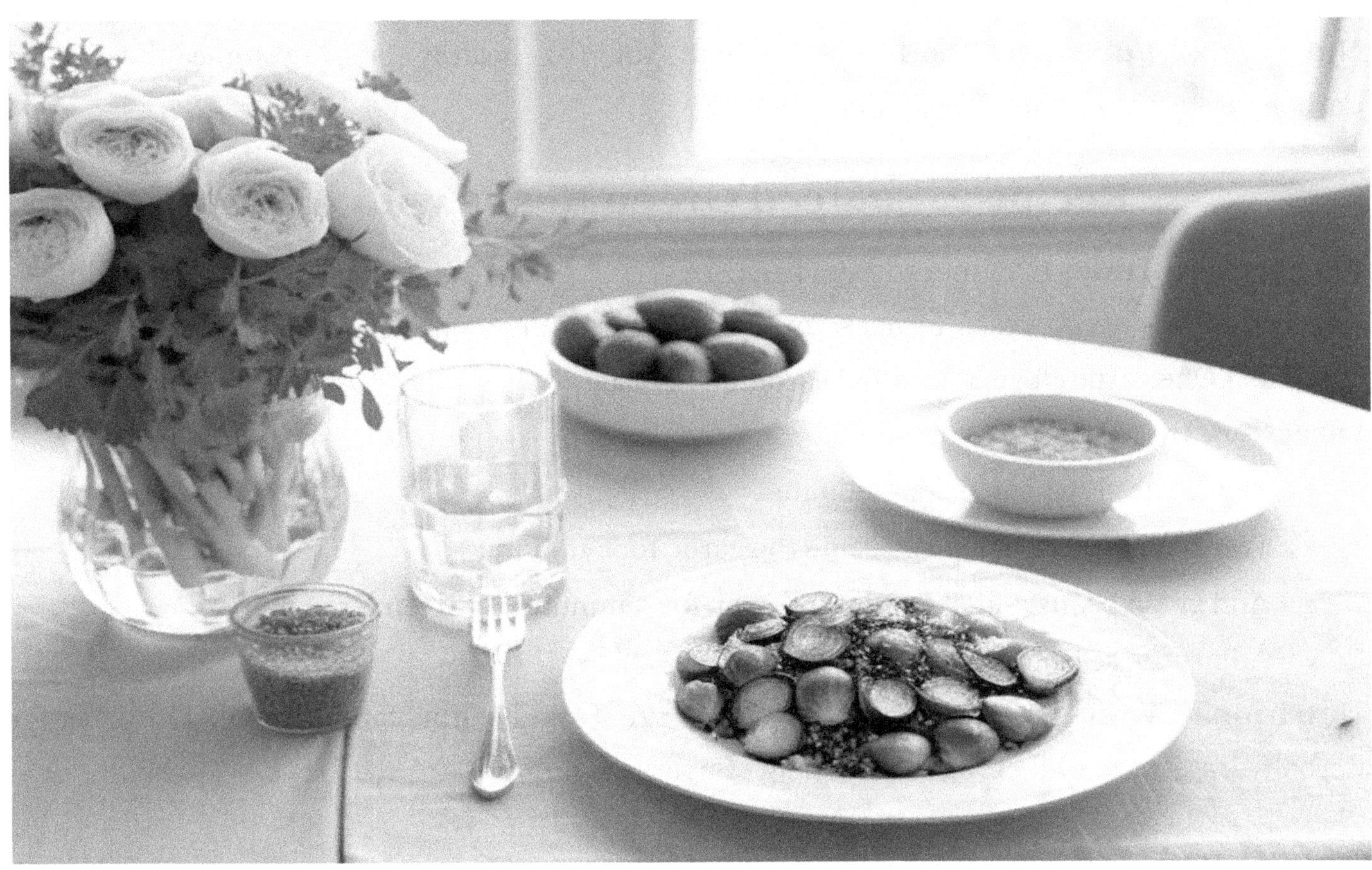

7.1: Vegetable Sides

Vegetables are essential to any diabetes-friendly diet, providing fiber, vitamins, and minerals. These vegetable-based side dishes are designed to be both nutritious and flavorful, ensuring you get the benefits of vegetables in various delicious forms. Enjoy these simple yet satisfying vegetable sides with your meals.

Recipe 1: Balsamic Glazed Roasted Brussels Sprouts

Preparation Time: 20 minutes | **Servings:** 1

Ingredients: • 1 cup Brussels sprouts, halved • One tablespoon of olive oil • One teaspoon of balsamic vinegar • Seasoning to taste

Directions:

- Heat the oven until it reaches 400°F (200°C).
- Coat the Brussels sprouts with a drizzle of olive oil, then season as desired.
- Roast for 15-20 minutes until crispy.
- Drizzle with balsamic vinegar and serve.

Nutritional Values: • Calories: 150 • Fat: 10g (9g healthy fats, 1g unhealthy fats) • Carbohydrates: 12g • Protein: 3g • Sugar: 3g

Recipe 2: Sautéed Green Beans with Almonds

Preparation Time: 15 minutes | **Servings:** 1

Ingredients: • 1 cup green beans • One tablespoon of olive oil • One tablespoon of slivered almonds • One garlic clove, minced • Seasoning to taste

Directions:

- Steam the green beans for 5 minutes.
- Warm olive oil in a pan and sauté the garlic for 1 minute.
- Add green beans and almonds, and cook for 5 minutes until tender.
- Adjust the seasoning to taste, then serve.

Nutritional Values: • Calories: 180 • Fat: 12g (10g healthy fats, 2g unhealthy fats) • Carbohydrates: 12g • Fiber: 6g • Protein: 4g • Sugar: 2g

Recipe 3: Garlic Mashed Cauliflower

Preparation Time: 15 minutes | **Servings:** 1

Ingredients: • 1/2 head cauliflower, chopped • One tablespoon of olive oil • One garlic clove, minced • Seasoning to taste

Directions:

- Simmer the cauliflower for about 10 minutes until tender.
- Drain and mash with olive oil and garlic.
- Sprinkle with a bit of seasoning, and enjoy while hot.

Nutritional Values: • Calories: 130 • Fat: 9g (8g healthy fats, 1g unhealthy fats) • Carbohydrates: 10g • Fiber: 5g • Protein: 3g• Sugar: 2g

Recipe 4: Grilled Zucchini with Parmesan

Preparation Time: 10 minutes | **Servings:** 1

Ingredients: • One small zucchini, sliced • One teaspoon of olive oil • One tablespoon grated Parmesan cheese • Seasoning to taste

Directions:

- Drizzle olive oil on the zucchini slices and season.
- Grill for 5 minutes on each side until tender.
- Sprinkle with Parmesan and serve.

Nutritional Values: • Calories: 120 • Fat: 8g (7g healthy fats, 1g unhealthy fats) • Carbohydrates: 6g • Fiber: 2g • Protein: 5g • Sugar: 2g

Recipe 5: Roasted Carrots with Thyme

Preparation Time: 20 minutes | **Servings:** 1

Ingredients: • 1 cup baby carrots • One teaspoon of olive oil • 1/2 teaspoon of dried thyme • Seasoning to taste

Directions:

- Heat the oven until it reaches 400°F (200°C).
- Toss the carrots with olive oil, thyme, and seasoning.
- Cook in the oven for 20 minutes until they become tender and develop a caramelized exterior.

Nutritional Values: • Calories: 100 • Fat: 5g (4g healthy fats, 1g unhealthy fats) • Carbohydrates: 12g • Fiber: 4g • Protein: 1g • Sugar: 6g

7.2: Whole Grains and Legumes

Whole grains and legumes are full of fiber and essential nutrients, making them excellent for a diabetes-friendly diet. These side dishes are designed to be filling and nutritious, helping to maintain steady blood sugar and adding heartiness and flavor to any meal.

Recipe 1: Quinoa Pilaf with Herbs

Preparation Time: 15 minutes | **Servings:** 1

Ingredients: • 1/4 cup quinoa • 1/2 cup vegetable broth • One tablespoon of chopped parsley • One teaspoon of olive oil • Salt and pepper

Directions:

- Wash the quinoa, then simmer in vegetable broth for 15 minutes.
- Mix the mixture with a fork, incorporating olive oil, parsley, salt, and pepper. Serve immediately.

Nutritional Values: • Calories: 180 • Fat: 6g (5g healthy fats, 1g unhealthy fats) • Carbohydrates: 25g • Fiber: 5g • Protein: 6g • Sugar: 1g

Recipe 2: Lentil Salad with Cucumber and Tomato

Preparation Time: 15 minutes | **Servings:** 1

Ingredients: • 1/4 cup of cooked lentils • 1/4 of cucumber, diced • 1/4 cup of cherry tomatoes, cut in half • One teaspoon of olive oil • One teaspoon of lemon juice • Salt and pepper

Directions:

- Combine lentils, cucumber, and tomatoes in a bowl.
- Pour olive oil and lemon juice, sprinkle with salt and pepper, and mix well.

Nutritional Values: • Calories: 160 • Fat: 6g (5g healthy fats, 1g unhealthy fats) • Carbohydrates: 22g • Fiber: 9g • Protein: 7g • Sugar: 2g

Recipe 3: Brown Rice with Garlic and Spinach

Preparation Time: 20 minutes | **Servings:** 1

Ingredients: • 1/4 cup brown rice • 1/2 cup fresh spinach • One garlic clove, minced • One teaspoon of olive oil • Salt and pepper

Directions:

- Prepare the brown rice following the instructions on the package.
- Cook the garlic and spinach in olive oil until they soften and wilt.
- Stir the spinach into the rice, add a dash of seasoning, then serve.

Nutritional Values: • Calories: 200 • Fat: 5g (4g healthy fats, 1g unhealthy fats) • Carbohydrates: 35g • Fiber: 4g • Protein: 5g • Sugar: 1g

Recipe 4: Barley with Mushrooms

Preparation Time: 30 minutes | **Servings:** 1

Ingredients: • 1/4 cup of pearl barley • 1/4 cup mushrooms, sliced • One tablespoon of olive oil • 1/2 teaspoon of thyme • Salt and pepper

Directions:

- Cook barley in water for 25 minutes until tender.
- Sauté mushrooms in a bit of olive oil for 5 minutes.
- Stir in the cooked barley, thyme, salt, and pepper. Serve immediately.

Nutritional Values: • Calories: 220 • Fat: 8g (7g healthy fats, 1g unhealthy fats) • Carbohydrates: 35g • Fiber: 8g • Protein: 6g • Sugar: 2g

Recipe 5: Chickpea and Red Pepper Stew

Preparation Time: 25 minutes | **Servings:** 1

Ingredients: • 1/2 cup of chickpeas, cooked • 1/4 of red bell pepper, chopped • 1/4 onion, chopped • One teaspoon spoonful of olive oil • 1/4 cup of low-sodium vegetable broth • Salt and pepper

Directions:

- Sauté onion and bell pepper in hot olive oil for around 5 minutes.
- Add chickpeas and vegetable broth and simmer for 10 minutes.
- Add a dash of salt and pepper, then serve.

Nutritional Values: • Calories: 210 • Fat: 6g (5g healthy fats, 1g unhealthy fats) • Carbohydrates: 32g • Fiber: 10g • Protein: 8g • Sugar: 4g

7.3: Creative Complements

Side dishes can be an exciting opportunity to get creative in the kitchen. These recipes combine unique flavors and textures to bring fresh life to your meals. Whether you're looking for something crunchy, tangy, or comforting, these creative side dishes will make your meals memorable and diabetes-friendly.

Recipe 1: Cucumber Salad with Yogurt and Dill

Preparation Time: 10 minutes | **Servings:** 1

Ingredients: • 1/2 cucumber, thinly sliced • Two tablespoons of plain Greek yogurt • One teaspoon of fresh dill chopped • One teaspoon of lemon juice • Salt and pepper.

Directions:

- Combine the cucumber, yogurt, dill, and lemon juice in a bowl.
- Gently mix, add some salt and pepper, and serve chilled.

Nutritional Values: • Calories: 80 • Fat: 3g (2g healthy fats, 1g unhealthy fats) • Carbohydrates: 7g • Fiber: 1g • Protein: 5g • Sugar: 3g

Recipe 2: Roasted Sweet Potato Wedges

Preparation Time: 25 minutes | **Servings:** 1

Ingredients: • One small sweet potato, cut into wedges • One teaspoon of olive oil • 1/2 teaspoon paprika • Salt and pepper.

Directions:

- Bring the oven to 400°F (200°C).
- Mix the sweet potato wedges with olive oil, paprika, salt, and pepper.
- Roast for 20-25 minutes until crispy.

Nutritional Values: • Calories: 180 • Fat: 5g (4g healthy fats, 1g unhealthy fats) • Carbohydrates: 30g • Fiber: 6g • Protein: 2g • Sugar: 8g

Recipe 3: Cauliflower Rice with Lime and Cilantro

Preparation Time: 10 minutes | **Servings:** 1

Ingredients: • 1 cup cauliflower rice (grated cauliflower) • One tablespoon of fresh cilantro, chopped • One teaspoon of lime juice • One teaspoon of olive oil • Salt and pepper

Directions:

- Cook the cauliflower rice in olive oil for about 5 minutes until it reaches the desired tenderness.
- Mix in lime juice and cilantro, then season to taste before serving.

Nutritional Values: • Calories: 90 • Fat: 5g (4g healthy fats, 1g unhealthy fats) • Carbohydrates: 9g • Fiber: 3g • Protein: 2g • Sugar: 3g

Recipe 4: Avocado and Tomato Salad

Preparation Time: 5 minutes | **Servings:** 1

Ingredients: • 1/4 avocado, diced • 1/2 tomato, finely chopped • One tablespoon of olive oil • One teaspoon of lemon juice • Salt and pepper

Directions:

- Mix avocado and tomato in a bowl.
- Finish by drizzling olive oil and a splash of lemon juice, then season to your liking.

Nutritional Values: • Calories: 140 • Fat: 12g (10g healthy fats, 2g unhealthy fats) Carbohydrates: 6g • Fiber: 4g • Protein: 2g • Sugar: 2g

Recipe 5: Baked Eggplant Rounds with Parmesan

Preparation Time: 20 minutes | **Servings:** 1

Ingredients: • 1/2 eggplant, sliced • One tablespoon of olive oil • One tablespoon of grated Parmesan cheese • Salt and pepper.

Directions:

- Heat the oven until it reaches 375°F (190°C).
- Rub olive oil onto the slices of eggplant, then season to your liking.
- After baking for a quarter of an hour, top with Parmesan and continue baking for five more minutes.

Nutritional Values: • Calories: 160 • Fat: 10g (9g healthy fats, 1g unhealthy fats) • Carbohydrates: 12g • Fiber: 5g • Protein: 4g • Sugar: 4g

Conclusion

Incorporating various side dishes in your meals is an enjoyable way to enhance flavor, texture, and nutrition while controlling Type 2 diabetes. These side dishes complement your main courses and provide essential nutrients like fiber, vitamins, and healthy fats that help support your overall health.

The recipes in this chapter are designed to be simple, versatile, and adaptable to your preferences. You can savor flavorful, satisfying meals by incorporating veggie sides, whole grains, beans, and inventive additions while managing your blood sugar effectively. Experimenting with side dishes offers an opportunity to discover new flavors and ingredients that make healthy eating exciting. Whether cooking for yourself or others, these recipes will help you create balanced and enjoyable meals. Remember that nutritious meals can be both tasty and satisfying, especially when you explore the wide range of side dishes that contribute to your overall health.

Chapter 8: Desserts

Introduction

For many, dessert is the ultimate comfort, a delightful conclusion to a meal, or a brief moment of indulgence. However, for individuals managing Type 2 diabetes, desserts can seem off-limits. However, this doesn't have to be the case. With thoughtful preparation and healthier ingredients, desserts can be part of a balanced diet. The key is creating diabetes-friendly sweets that satisfy your cravings without causing blood sugar spikes.

This chapter is dedicated to delicious dessert recipes that are low in sugar and packed with nutritious ingredients. From creamy delicacies and baked treats to fruity delights, these recipes will allow you to enjoy dessert while supporting your health objectives. Whether you crave something rich and chocolatey or light and fruity, there's a treat here for everyone.

An occasional sweet treat can be enjoyed without guilt or health concerns. These dessert recipes are designed with diabetes in mind so you can indulge in something delicious while maintaining control of your blood sugar. Let's explore these guilt-free desserts that allow you to savor every bite.

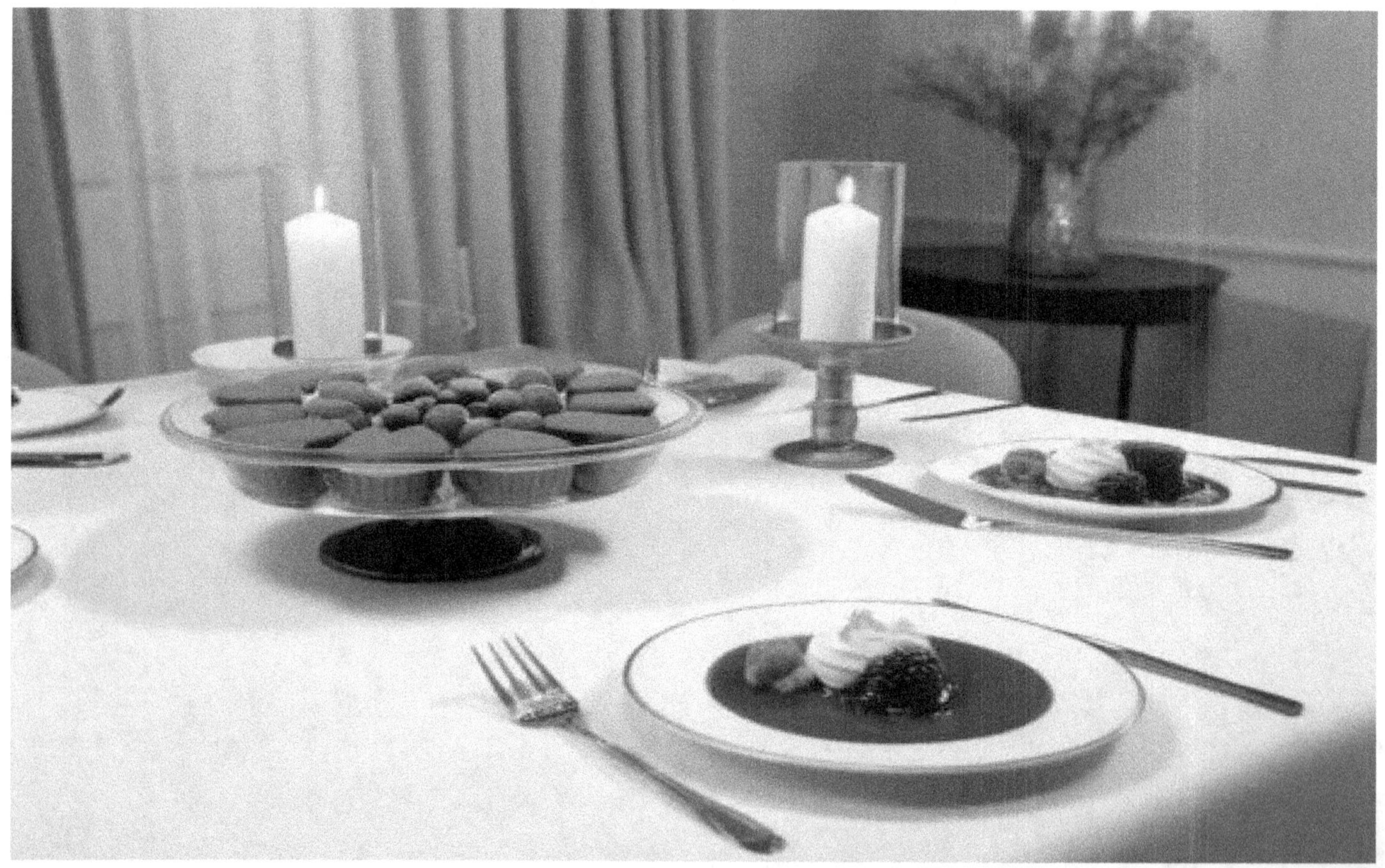

8.1: Sweet Treats Without the Guilt

You can still enjoy sweet treats even while managing diabetes. This section offers dessert recipes using healthier ingredients to satisfy your cravings while stabilizing blood sugar levels. These treats are light, flavorful, and designed to fit perfectly into a diabetes-friendly diet.

Recipe 1: Chocolate Avocado Mousse

Preparation Time: 10 minutes | **Servings:** 1

Ingredients: • 1/2 ripe avocado • One tablespoon of unsweetened cocoa powder • One teaspoon of stevia or sugar-free sweetener • 1/2 teaspoon of vanilla extract • A pinch of salt

Directions:

- Combine all the ingredients and blend until you achieve a smooth and creamy consistency.
- Chill it in the fridge for 30 minutes before serving.

Nutritional Values: • Calories: 180 • Fat: 14g (12g healthy fats, 2g unhealthy fats) • Carbohydrates: 10g • Fiber: 7g • Protein: 2g • Sugar: 2g

Recipe 2: Greek Yogurt with Cinnamon and Walnuts

Preparation Time: 5 minutes | **Servings:** 1

Ingredients: • 1/2 cup of unsweetened Greek yogurt • 1/2 teaspoon of ground cinnamon • One tablespoon of chopped walnuts • One teaspoon sugar-free sweetener (optional)

Directions:

- Mix the cinnamon into the yogurt.
- Top with walnuts and serve.

Nutritional Values: • Calories: 140 • Fat: 7g (6g healthy fats, 1g unhealthy fats) • Carbohydrates: 8g • Fiber: 2g • Protein: 12g • Sugar: 4g

Recipe 3: Coconut Chia Pudding

Preparation Time: 5 minutes (+ overnight chilling) | **Servings:** 1

Ingredients: • 1/4 cup unsweetened almond milk • One tablespoon of chia seeds • One tablespoon of unsweetened shredded coconut • One teaspoon of sugar-free sweetener

Directions:

- Mix all ingredients in a compact container.
- Refrigerate overnight to allow it to thicken. Stir well before serving.

Nutritional Values:• Calories: 130 • Fat: 9g (8g healthy fats, 1g unhealthy fats) • Carbohydrates: 8g • Fiber: 5g • Protein: 3g • Sugar: 1g

Recipe 4: Almond Butter Bites

Preparation Time: 5 minutes | **Servings:** 1

Ingredients: • One tablespoon of almond butter • One teaspoon of sugar-free sweetener • One tablespoon of rolled oats • 1/2 teaspoon of vanilla extract

Directions:
- Mix all ingredients.
- Form into small balls and chill for 15 minutes before serving.

Nutritional Values: • Calories: 110 • Fat: 9g (8g healthy fats, 1g unhealthy fats) • Carbohydrates: 6g • Fiber: 2g • Protein: 4g • Sugar: 1g

Recipe 5: Baked Apple with Cinnamon

Preparation Time: 20 minutes | **Servings:** 1

Ingredients: • One small apple • 1/2 teaspoon cinnamon • One teaspoon of sugar-free sweetener • One teaspoon of chopped almonds

Directions:
- Core the apple and sprinkle with cinnamon, sweetener, and almonds.
- Bake at 350°F (175°C) for 15-20 minutes until soft.

Nutritional Values: • Calories: 120 • Fat: 4g (3g healthy fats, 1g unhealthy fats) • Carbohydrates: 20g • Fiber: 5g • Protein: 2g • Sugar: 10g

8.2: Baking with Sugar Alternatives

Baking doesn't have to mean loading up on sugar. This section will explore desserts that use sugar alternatives to create lower-sugar baked goods. With the right ingredients, you can enjoy cookies, cakes, and more without worrying about your blood sugar levels.

Recipe 1: Almond Flour Cookies

Preparation Time: 15 minutes | **Servings:** 1

Ingredients: • Two tablespoons of almond flour • One teaspoon of coconut oil • One teaspoon of sugar-free sweetener • 1/4 teaspoon vanilla extract

Directions:

- Mix all ingredients.
- Mold into a cookie shape and bake at 350°F (175°C) for 10-12 minutes.

Nutritional Values: • Calories: 120 • Fat: 10g (9g healthy fats, 1g unhealthy fats) • Carbohydrates: 5g • Fiber: 2g • Protein: 3g • Sugar: 0g

Recipe 2: Low-Sugar Blueberry Muffin

Preparation Time: 25 minutes | **Servings:** 1

Ingredients: • Two tablespoons of almond flour • One tablespoon of fresh blueberries • One egg white • 1/2 teaspoon baking powder • One teaspoon of sugar-free sweetener

Directions:

- Mix the flour, egg white, baking powder, and sweetener.
- Fold in the blueberries and pour into a muffin mold.
- Bake at 350°F (175°C) for 20 minutes.

Nutritional Values: • Calories: 150 • Fat: 7g (6g healthy fats, 1g unhealthy fats) • Carbohydrates: 10g • Fiber: 4g • Protein: 6g • Sugar: 2g

Recipe 3: Sugar-Free Brownie Mug Cake

Preparation Time: 5 minutes | **Servings:** 1

Ingredients: • One tablespoon of almond flour • One tablespoon of unsweetened cocoa powder • One teaspoon of sugar-free sweetener • One egg white • 1/4 teaspoon of vanilla extract

Directions:

- Place all the ingredients into a microwave-safe mug, ensuring they are thoroughly mixed.
- Set the microwave to high and cook for 1 minute.

Nutritional Values: • Calories: 140 • Fat: 9g (8g healthy fats, 1g unhealthy fats) • Carbohydrates: 7g • Fiber: 3g • Protein: 5g • Sugar: 1g

Recipe 4: Coconut Flour Pancake

Preparation Time:10 minutes | **Servings:** 1

Ingredients: • One tablespoon of coconut flour • One egg • One tablespoon of unsweetened almond milk • One teaspoon of sugar-free sweetener

Directions:

- Mix all ingredients until smooth.
- Cook on a hot, lightly greased skillet for 2-3 minutes on each side.

Nutritional Values: • Calories: 130 • Fat: 8g (7g healthy fats, 1g unhealthy fats) • Carbohydrates: 6g • Fiber: 3g • Protein: 6g • Sugar: 1g

Recipe 5: Sugar-Free Lemon Bars

Preparation Time: 30 minutes | **Servings:** 1

Ingredients: • Two tablespoons of almond flour • One teaspoon of coconut oil • One egg white • One tablespoon of lemon juice • One teaspoon of sugar-free sweetener

Directions:

- Mix the almond flour and coconut oil to form a crust, and bake for 10 minutes at 350°F (175°C).
- Whisk the egg white, lemon juice, and sweetener, and pour over the crust.
- Bake for another 15 minutes.

Nutritional Values: • Calories: 140 • Fat: 10g (8g healthy fats, 2g unhealthy fats) • Carbohydrates: 8g • Fiber: 3g • Protein: 4g • Sugar: 1g

8.3: Fruity Favorites

Fruits are nature's candy, offering natural sweetness, essential vitamins, and fiber. In this section, we'll explore simple and delightful desserts that use fruits as the star ingredient, keeping sugar content lower while providing a burst of flavor.

Recipe 1: Berry Parfait

Preparation Time: 5 minutes | **Servings:** 1

Ingredients: • 1/4 cup mixed berries (blueberries, raspberries) • Two tablespoons of plain Greek yogurt • One teaspoon of chia seeds • 1/2 teaspoon honey (optional)

Directions:

- Layer the berries and yogurt in a glass.
- Add some chia seeds and, if you want, some honey.

Nutritional Values: • Calories: 110 • Fat: 4g (3g healthy fats, 1g unhealthy fats) • Carbohydrates: 12g • Fiber: 4g • Protein: 6g • Sugar: 6g

Recipe 2: Grilled Peaches with Ricotta

Preparation Time: 10 minutes | **Servings:** 1

Ingredients: • One small peach, halved • One tablespoon of ricotta cheese • 1/2 teaspoon honey (optional)

Directions:

- Grill the peach halves for 5 minutes until tender.
- Top with ricotta and drizzle with honey if desired.

Nutritional Values: • Calories: 90 • Fat: 4g (3g healthy fats, 1g unhealthy fats) • Carbohydrates: 12g • Fiber: 2g • Protein: 3g • Sugar: 9g

Recipe 3: Frozen Banana Bites

Preparation Time: 5 minutes (+ freezing) | **Servings:** 1

Ingredients: • 1/2 banana, sliced • One tablespoon of peanut butter • One tablespoon of unsweetened shredded coconut

Directions:

- Spread peanut butter on each banana slice.
- Coat with shredded coconut and freeze for an hour

Nutritional Values: • Calories: 120 • Fat: 7g (6g healthy fats, 1g unhealthy fats) • Carbohydrates: 15g • Fiber: 3g • Protein: 3g • Sugar: 8g

Recipe 4: Apple and Cinnamon Compote

Preparation Time: 10 minutes | **Servings:** 1

Ingredients: • One small apple, peeled and chopped • 1/2 teaspoon cinnamon • One teaspoon water • One teaspoon of sugar-free sweetener.

Directions:

- Cook the apple, cinnamon, water, and sweetener in a small pot for 10 minutes until soft.
- It can be served warm or chilled.

Nutritional Values: • Calories: 80 • Fat: 0g • Carbohydrates: 20g • Fiber: 4g • Protein: 0g • Sugar: 12g

Recipe 5: Kiwi and Strawberry Salad

Preparation Time: 5 minutes | **Servings:** 1

Ingredients: • 1/2 kiwi, peeled and thinly sliced • 1/4 cup strawberries, halved • One tablespoon of fresh mint, chopped

Directions:

- Mix the kiwi and strawberries in a bowl.
- Top with chopped mint and serve.

Nutritional Values: • Calories: 50 • Fat: 0g • Carbohydrates: 12g • Fiber: 3g • Protein: 1g • Sugar: 9g

Conclusion

Desserts can be a delightful part of life, even for diabetes patients. The key is to make thoughtful choices, focusing on healthier ingredients and natural sweetness. The recipes in this chapter are crafted to curb your sweet cravings while maintaining steady blood sugar levels. You can enjoy indulgent treats without worrying by using sugar alternatives, incorporating fruits, and choosing nutritious ingredients.

The delight of dessert lies in the joy and satisfaction it brings to the conclusion of a meal. With these diabetes-friendly recipes, you can enjoy sweet treats guilt-free. Whether it's a chocolatey mousse, a fruity parfait, or a warm baked treat, there are numerous choices to explore and enjoy. Remember, balance is critical. You don't need to deny yourself the pleasure of dessert. Still, by making intelligent choices, you can include these sweet moments in your diabetes management plan. We hope these recipes inspire you to get creative and enjoy desserts as a component of a nutritious, fulfilling lifestyle.

Chapter 9: Drinks and Smoothies

Introduction

For individuals over 50 managing diabetes, keeping well-hydrated is crucial for overall wellness and controlling blood sugar levels. Choosing the right drinks can prevent blood sugar spikes, keep energy steady, and support metabolism. Plenty of low-sugar, low-calorie options make it easy to enjoy beverages that positively affect diabetes management. This chapter presents a wide array of refreshing, nutritious drinks tailored explicitly for people with diabetes. From hydrating, blood-sugar-friendly beverages to calming herbal teas and nutrient-dense smoothies, these recipes offer diverse flavors and health benefits. Each recipe is crafted to support hydration, energy, and healthy blood sugar levels. Dive in and find new favorites to make hydration both enjoyable and beneficial.

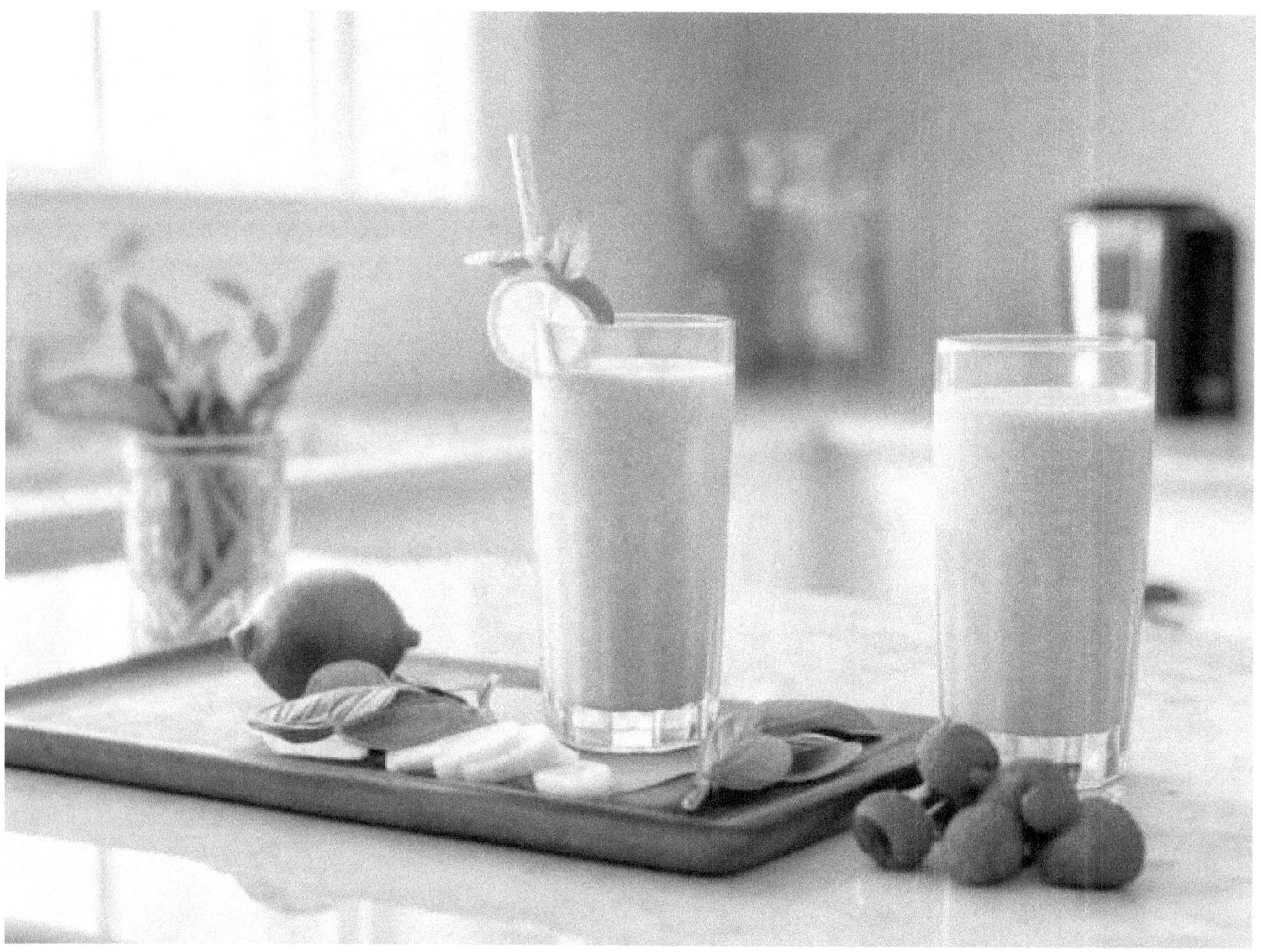

9.1 Healthy Beverages

This section offers a diverse selection of five refreshing drink recipes that are light on sugar, rich in flavor, and perfect for maintaining hydration and energy levels. Each recipe is a unique and delicious option for those looking to support their blood sugar balance and metabolic health.

Recipe 1: Citrus Basil Infusion

Preparation Time: 5 minutes | **Servings:** 1

Ingredients: • 1/2 lemon, sliced • 1/2 lime, sliced • 3-4 fresh basil leaves • One cup cold water • Ice cubes

Preparation Method: Combine lemon, lime, and basil with water and ice in a glass.

Directions: Stir well and enjoy immediately.

Tips & Suggestions: Basil adds antioxidants, which may help regulate blood sugar.

Nutritional Values: • Calories: 10 • Fat: 0g • Carbohydrates: 3g • Fiber: 1g • Protein: 0g • Sugar: 1g

Recipe 2: Apple Cider Vinegar Refresher

Preparation Time: 5 minutes | **Servings:** 1

Ingredients: • One tablespoon apple cider vinegar • One cup cold water • 1/2 teaspoon cinnamon • Ice cubes

Preparation Method: Mix apple cider vinegar and cinnamon in a glass with water.

Directions: Add ice cubes and enjoy chilled.

Tips & Suggestions: Cinnamon may aid in blood sugar control and add flavor without sugar.

Nutritional Values: • Calories: 5 • Fat: 0g • Carbohydrates: 1g • Fiber: 0g • Protein: 0g • Sugar: 0g

Recipe 3: Cucumber Mint Cooler

Preparation Time: 5 minutes | **Servings:** 1

Ingredients: • 1/2 cucumber, thinly sliced • 2-3 fresh mint leaves • One cup water • Ice cubes

Preparation Method: Combine cucumber and mint in a glass with water and ice.

Directions: Stir well and enjoy.

Tips & Suggestions: Mint adds freshness and may aid in digestion.

Nutritional Values: • Calories: 5 • Fat: 0g • Carbohydrates: 2g • Fiber: 0g • Protein: 0g • Sugar: 1g

Recipe 4: Berry Lime Sparkler

Preparation Time: 5 minutes | **Servings:** 1

Ingredients: • 1/4 cup mixed berries (blueberries, raspberries) • Juice of 1/2 lime • One cup sparkling water • Ice cubes

Preparation Method: Muddle berries in a glass and incorporate a hint of lime juice followed by a touch of sparkling water.

Directions: Add ice and enjoy.

Tips & Suggestions: This drink contains antioxidants and benefits overall health.

Nutritional Values: • Calories: 20 • Fat: 0g • Carbohydrates: 5g • Fiber: 1g • Protein: 0g • Sugar: 3g

Recipe 5: Green Tea Lemonade

Preparation Time: 10 minutes | **Servings:** 1

Ingredients: • One cup brewed green tea, cooled • Juice of 1/2 lemon • 1-2 teaspoons of honey or a few drops of stevia (optional) • Ice cubes

Preparation Method: Combine green tea, lemon juice, and optional sweetener in a glass.

Directions: Add ice and enjoy.

Tips & Suggestions: Green tea is known for its antioxidants and potential blood sugar benefits.

Nutritional Values: • Calories: 25 (with honey) • Fat: 0g • Carbohydrates: 6g • Fiber: 0g • Protein: 0g • Sugar: 4g

9.2 Herbal Teas and Infusions

Herbal teas offer a warm, soothing way to stay hydrated, relax, and gain health benefits without added sugars or calories. These recipes provide diabetes-friendly options for winding down and staying hydrated all day.

Recipe 1: Chamomile Lavender Tea

Preparation Time: 5 minutes | **Servings:** 1

Ingredients: • 1 teaspoon of chamomile • 1/2 teaspoon of lavender • One cup of freshly boiled water

Preparation Method:

Steep chamomile and lavender in freshly boiled water for five minutes.

Strain and enjoy.

Tips & Suggestions: Chamomile may help improve sleep quality.

Nutritional Values: • Calories: 0 • Fat: 0g • Carbohydrates: 0g • Fiber: 0g • Protein: 0g • Sugar: 0g

Recipe 2: Ginger Turmeric Infusion

Preparation Time: 10 minutes | **Servings:** 1

Ingredients:• 1-inch piece fresh ginger, sliced • 1/2 teaspoon turmeric powder • One cup freshly boiled water

Preparation Method:

1. Infuse ginger and turmeric in freshly boiled water for five minutes.
2. Drain and enjoy the infusion.

Tips & Suggestions: Turmeric has anti-inflammatory benefits.

Nutritional Values:• Calories: 5 • Fat: 0g • Carbohydrates: 1g • Fiber: 0g • Protein: 0g • Sugar: 0g

Recipe 3: Peppermint Fennel Tea

Preparation Time: 5 minutes | **Servings:** 1

Ingredients:•: 1 teaspoon peppermint leaves • 1/2 teaspoon fennel seeds • One cup of freshly boiled water.

Preparation Method:

1. Steep peppermint and fennel seeds in freshly boiled water for five minutes.
2. Drain and enjoy the tea.

Tips & Suggestions: Fennel is appreciated for its digestive benefits.

Nutritional Values: • Calories: 0 • Fat: 0g • Carbohydrates: 0g • Fiber: 0g • Protein: 0g • Sugar: 0g

Recipe 4: Lemon Verbena Soother

Preparation Time: 5 minutes | **Servings:** 1

Ingredients: One teaspoon of lemon verbena leaves • One cup of freshly boiled water.

Preparation Method:

1. Steep lemon verbena in freshly boiled water for five minutes.
2. Filter and enjoy.

Tips & Suggestions: Lemon verbena is celebrated for its relaxing qualities and ability to aid digestion.

Nutritional Values: • Calories: 0 • Fat: 0g • Carbohydrates: 0g • Fiber: 0g • Protein: 0g • Sugar: 0g

Recipe 5: Rooibos Cinnamon Tea

Preparation Time: 5 minutes | **Servings:** 1

Ingredients: • 1 teaspoon rooibos tea • 1/4 teaspoon cinnamon • One cup freshly boiled water

Preparation Method:

1. Steep rooibos tea and cinnamon in freshly boiled water for five minutes.
2. Filter and enjoy.

Tips & Suggestions: Cinnamon adds a natural sweetness that may help control blood sugar.

Nutritional Values: • Calories: 5 • Fat: 0g • Carbohydrates: 1g • Fiber: 0g • Protein: 0g • Sugar: 0g

9.3 Nutritional Smoothies

Smoothies are a fantastic option for packing essential nutrients, fiber, and antioxidants. They serve as a perfect snack or meal replacement for individuals over 50 managing diabetes. The best recipes use low-GI fruits, protein, and fiber while avoiding added sugars, aiding in the stability of blood glucose levels.

Recipe 1: Berry Almond Smoothie

Preparation Time: 5 minutes | **Servings:** 1

Ingredients: • 1/2 cup mixed berries (blueberries, strawberries) • 1/2 cup of almond milk without added sugars • 1 tablespoon chia seeds • 1/4 cup Greek yogurt (without added sugars)

Preparation Method: Blend all ingredients until smooth.

Directions: Savor immediately after pouring into your preferred mug.

Tips & Suggestions: Chia seeds contribute essential nutrients and healthy fats that aid digestion and stabilize blood sugar.

Nutritional Values: • Calories: 150 • Fat: 5g (3g healthy fats) • Carbohydrates: 18g • Fiber: 6g • Protein: 8g • Sugar: 7g (natural sugars)

Recipe 2: Green Power Smoothie

Preparation Time: 5 minutes | **Servings:** 1

Ingredients: • 1/2 cup with spinach • 1/2 small green apple, chopped • 1/2 cup cucumber, chopped • 1/2 cup coconut water with no added sugars • 1 tablespoon of ground flaxseeds

Preparation Method: Blend all ingredients until smooth.

Directions: Savor immediately after pouring into your preferred mug.

Tips & Suggestions: Adding spinach and flaxseeds gives this smoothie extra fiber, which is excellent for controlling blood sugar.

Nutritional Values: • Calories: 90 • Fat: 2g (1.5g healthy fats) • Carbohydrates: 15g • Fiber: 5g • Protein: 2g • Sugar: 7g

Recipe 3: Avocado Cocoa Smoothie

Preparation Time: 5 minutes | **Servings:** 1

Ingredients: • 1/4 avocado • 1 tablespoon unsweetened cocoa powder • 1/2 cup almond milk (without added sugars) • 1/4 teaspoon vanilla extract • Ice cubes (optional)

Preparation Method: Blend all ingredients until they become smooth and creamy.

Directions: Savor immediately after pouring into your preferred mug.

Tips & Suggestions: This luscious, chocolatey smoothie is loaded with healthy fats, perfect for steady blood sugar levels.

Nutritional Values: • Calories: 120 • Fat: 8g (7g healthy fats) • Carbohydrates: 9g • Fiber: 5g • Protein: 2g • Sugar: 2g

Recipe 4: Tropical Ginger Smoothie

Preparation Time: 5 minutes | **Servings:** 1

Ingredients: • 1/4 cup pineapple, diced • 1/4 cup mango, diced • 1/2 cup unsweetened coconut milk • 1/4 teaspoon grated fresh ginger • Ice cubes (optional)

Preparation Method: Blend all ingredients until smooth.

Directions: Savor immediately after pouring into your preferred mug.

Tips & Suggestions: Ginger imparts a subtle warmth and can support digestion and blood sugar regulation.

Nutritional Values: • Calories: 130 • Fat: 4g (healthy fats from coconut milk) • Carbohydrates: 20g • Fiber: 3g • Protein: 1g • Sugar: 15g (natural sugars)

Recipe 5: Peanut Butter Banana Smoothie

Preparation Time: 5 minutes | **Servings:** 1

Ingredients: • 1/2 small banana • 1 tablespoon natural peanut butter (without added sugar) • 1/2 cup of almond milk (without added sugar) • 1/4 cup Greek yogurt (without added sugar) • Ice cubes (optional)

Preparation Method: Blend all ingredients until they reach a smooth and creamy consistency.

Directions: Savor immediately after pouring into your preferred mug.

Tips & Suggestions: This smoothie offers essential nutrients like proteins, beneficial fats, and fiber, making it a filling choice supporting blood sugar control.

Nutritional Values: • Calories: 180 • Fat: 7g (6g healthy fats) • Carbohydrates: 20g • Fiber: 4g • Protein: 8g • Sugar: 9g (natural sugars)

Conclusion

Beverages support diabetes management by offering hydration, energy, and nourishment. Incorporating these beverages into your routine allows you to enjoy delicious flavors while contributing to better blood sugar control and overall health. Experiment with these recipes and adapt them to your tastes. Each drink is crafted to be diabetes-friendly, easy to make, and beneficial for your wellness journey. Remember, staying hydrated and choosing nutritious beverages is essential to maintaining balance and living well with diabetes. Cheers to your health!

Chapter 10: Special Occasion Meals

Introduction

Special occasions bring joy and connection, often centered around shared meals. Cooking and sharing meals is vital to these moments, whether a holiday celebration, family gathering, or entertaining friends. Managing Type 2 diabetes can make enjoying meals feel challenging at times. Still, it's possible to savor delicious dishes with suitable recipes without compromising health goals. It is possible to create tasty, diabetes-friendly dishes that allow everyone to indulge while being mindful of their nutritional needs.

This chapter provides flavorful and nutritious recipes for special occasions, emphasizing maintaining blood sugar control while enjoying festive meals. From holiday-inspired recipes to tips for hosting diabetes-friendly gatherings, you'll find that celebrating with food doesn't have to mean sacrificing health. These recipes achieve an ideal balance by emphasizing whole ingredients, reducing unhealthy fats and added sugars, and enhancing flavor with herbs, spices, and nutrient-dense foods. Whether preparing a holiday feast, throwing a party, or enjoying a meal with your family, these recipes will guide you in creating satisfying dishes and being mindful of diabetes management. Let's explore how you can enjoy and feel good about indulging in delicious, balanced meals during special moments without guilt.

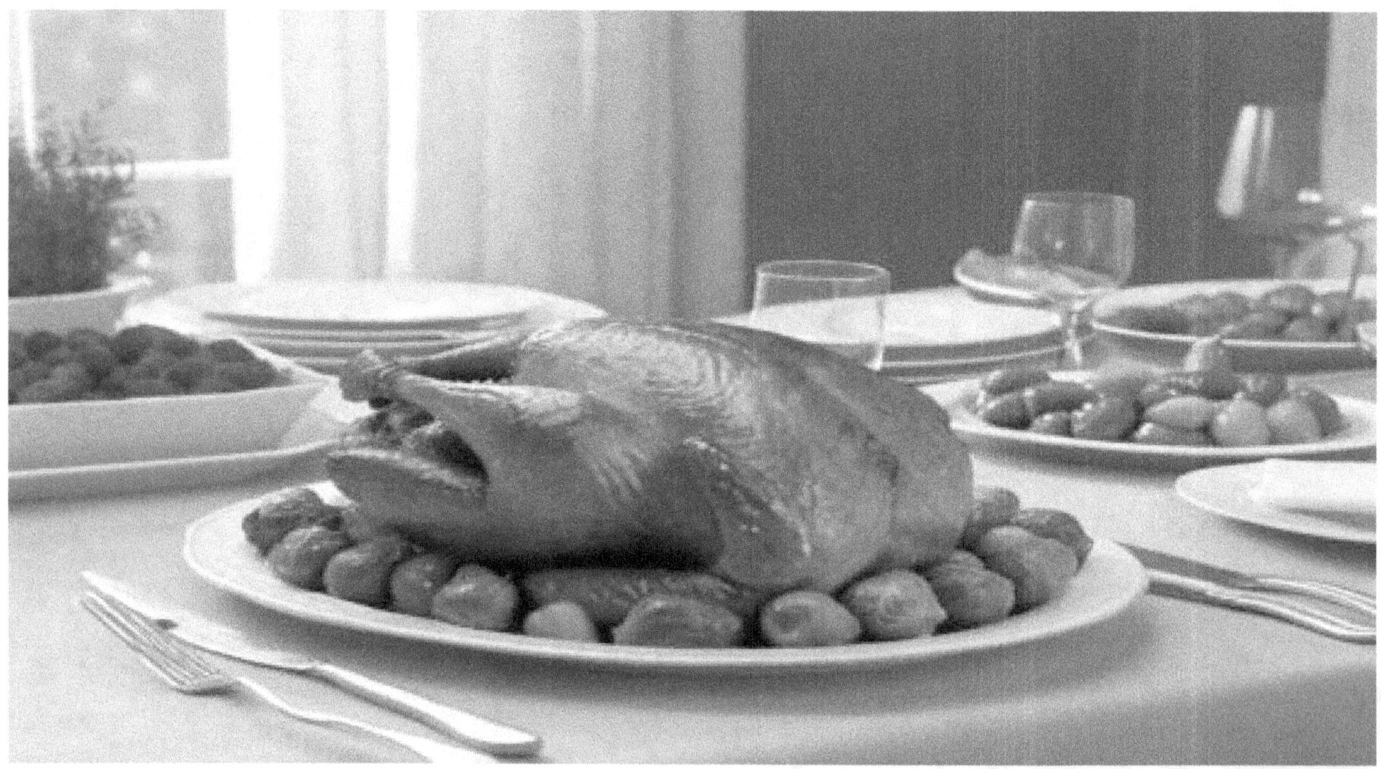

10.1: Holiday Recipes

Holidays are a time for celebration, where meals are vital in uniting people. These holiday recipes are designed to be festive, flavorful, and diabetes-friendly, allowing everyone to join in the celebrations. These dishes focus on balance, combining traditional flavors with ingredients that support good health.

Recipe 1: Herb-Roasted Turkey Breast

Preparation Time: 45 minutes | **Servings:** 1

Ingredients: • One small turkey breast (about 4 oz) • One teaspoon of olive oil • 1/2 teaspoon dried thyme • 1/2 teaspoon dried rosemary • Salt and pepper to taste

Preparation Method: Roasting

Directions:

- Bring the oven to 350°F (175°C).
- Rub olive oil, thyme, rosemary, salt, and pepper all over the turkey breast.
- Roast for 35-40 minutes until the internal temperature reaches 165°F (74°C).
- Let it rest for 5 minutes before you slice and serve it.

Tips & Suggestions: Serve the turkey with roasted vegetables or a fresh salad to create a nutritious and tasty meal.

Nutritional Values: • Calories: 220 • Fat: 8g (6g healthy fats, 2g unhealthy fats) • Carbohydrates: 1g • Fiber: 0g • Protein: 32g • Sugar: 0g

Recipe 2: Roasted Butternut Squash

Preparation Time: 30 minutes | **Servings:** 1

Ingredients: • 1 cup butternut squash, cubed • One teaspoon of olive oil • 1/2 teaspoon cinnamon • Salt and pepper to taste

Preparation Method: Roasting

Directions:

- Bring the oven to 400°F (200°C).
- Coat the squash in olive oil, cinnamon, salt, and pepper.
- Bake for 25-30 minutes until the squash becomes tender and caramelized.

Nutritional Values: • Calories: 90 • Fat: 3g (2g healthy fats, 1g unhealthy fats) • Carbohydrates: 18g • Fiber: 4g • Protein: 1g • Sugar: 4g

Recipe 3: Balsamic-Glazed Brussels Sprouts

Preparation Time: 25 minutes | **Servings**: 1

Ingredients: • 1 cup Brussels sprouts, halved • One teaspoon of balsamic vinegar • One teaspoon of olive oil • Salt and pepper to taste

Preparation Method: Roasting

Directions:

- Bring the oven to 400°F (200°C).
- Begin by adding Brussels sprouts to a mixing bowl. Lightly coat olive oil and balsamic vinaigrette, then season season to your liking with salt and pepper.
- Mix until everything is evenly covered.
- Roast for 20-25 minutes until tender, with crispy edges.

Tips & Suggestions: Serve the turkey with roasted vegetables or a fresh salad to create a nutritious and tasty meal

Nutritional Values: • Calories: 110 • Fat: 4g (3g healthy fats, 1g unhealthy fats) • Carbohydrates: 15g • Fiber: 6g • Protein: 3g • Sugar: 4g

Recipe 4: Cranberry-Orange Relish

Preparation Time: 10 minutes | **Servings**: 1

Ingredients: • 1/4 cup fresh cranberries • One tablespoon of fresh orange juice • 1/2 teaspoon stevia (or sugar-free sweetener)

Preparation Method: Blending

Directions:

- Blend the cranberries, orange juice, and stevia until smooth in a blender or food processor.
- Enjoy chilled or at room temperature as a delightful complement to your holiday meal.

Nutritional Values: • Calories: 40 • Fat: 0g • Carbohydrates: 10g • Fiber: 2g • Protein: 0g • Sugar: 3g

Recipe 5: Garlic Mashed Cauliflower

Preparation Time: 15 minutes | **Servings:** 1

Ingredients: • 1/2 head cauliflower, chopped • One clove of garlic, minced • One teaspoon of olive oil • Salt and pepper

Preparation Method: Boiling and mashing

Directions:

- Boil the cauliflower for 10 minutes until it softens.
- Drain and mash with olive oil, garlic, salt, and pepper.
- Use this as a nutritious substitute for mashed potatoes.

Nutritional Values: • Calories: 90 • Fat: 4g (3g healthy fats, 1g unhealthy fats) • Carbohydrates: 10g • Fiber: 3g • Protein: 2g • Sugar: 2g

10.2: Entertaining with Diabetes

Entertaining can be a joyful experience, and when managing diabetes, it's essential to serve dishes that cater to all tastes while keeping health in mind. This section offers balanced, flavorful recipes that are perfect for gatherings. These tips and recipes will ensure your guests are satisfied without compromising health.

Recipe 1: Caprese Skewers

Preparation Time: 10 minutes | **Servings**: 1

Ingredients: • Four cherry tomatoes • Two mini mozzarella balls • Two fresh basil leaves • One teaspoon of balsamic vinegar

Preparation Method: Assembling

Directions:

- Skewer the cherry tomatoes, mozzarella, and basil leaves.
- Please give it a balsamic vinegar splash and serve as a refreshing appetizer.

Nutritional Values:• Calories: 80 • Fat: 5g (4g healthy fats, 1g unhealthy fats) • Carbohydrates: 4g • Fiber: 1g • Protein: 4g • Sugar: 2g

Recipe 2: Stuffed Mini Peppers

Preparation Time: 15 minutes | **Servings**: 1

Ingredients: • Two mini bell peppers, halved and deseeded • One tablespoon of hummus • One teaspoon of chopped parsley

Preparation Method: Stuffing

Directions:

- Fill each pepper half with hummus.
- Garnish with parsley and serve chilled.

Nutritional Values: • Calories: 60 • Fat: 3g (2g healthy fats, 1g unhealthy fats) • Carbohydrates: 7g • Fiber: 2g • Protein: 2g • Sugar: 3g

Recipe 3: Zucchini Fritters

Preparation Time: 20 minutes | **Servings**: 1

Ingredients: • One small zucchini, grated • One egg white • One tablespoon of almond flour • Salt and pepper • One teaspoon of olive oil

Preparation Method: Frying

Directions:

- Mix the grated zucchini, egg white, almond flour, salt, and pepper.
- Gently spoon the mixture into a hot pan with olive oil.
- Cook until each side is golden brown, which should take approximately 3 minutes per side.

Nutritional Values: • Calories: 140 • Fat: 6g (5g healthy fats, 1g unhealthy fats) • Carbohydrates: 10g • Fiber: 3g • Protein: 5g • Sugar: 2g

Recipe 4: Grilled Chicken Bites with Avocado Dip

Preparation Time: 20 minutes | **Servings**: 1

Ingredients: • Four small chicken breast cubes • 1/4 avocado, mashed • One teaspoon of lemon juice • Salt and pepper

Preparation Method: Grilling

Directions:

- Season chicken cubes with your preferred spices. Grill for 3-4 minutes per side.
- Mix avocado with lemon juice to make the dip.

- Serve chicken bites with avocado dip on the side.

Nutritional Values: • Calories: 180 • Fat: 10g (9g healthy fats, 1g unhealthy fats) • Carbohydrates: 3g • Fiber: 2g • Protein: 20g • Sugar: 0g

Recipe 5: Cucumber and Salmon Bites

Preparation Time: 10 minutes | **Servings**: 1

Ingredients: • Four cucumber slices • 1 ounce smoked salmon • One teaspoon of cream cheese (optional) • Fresh dill for garnish

Preparation Method: Assembling

Directions:

- Gently coat each cucumber slice with a thin layer of cream cheese.
- Finish by adding a slice of smoked salmon and garnishing with fresh dill.

Nutritional Values: • Calories: 90 • Fat: 5g (4g healthy fats, 1g unhealthy fats) • Carbohydrates: 3g • Fiber: 1g • Protein: 8g • Sugar: 1g

10.3: Family Gatherings

Family meals bring everyone together; these recipes are designed to please diabetics and non-diabetics alike. With their perfect balance of flavors, these dishes are great for sharing. They will ensure everyone enjoys a wholesome and delicious meal that promotes health and connection.

Recipe 1: Baked Chicken Thigh with Rosemary

Preparation Time: 35 minutes | **Servings**: 1

Ingredients: • One chicken thigh, skinless • One teaspoon of olive oil • 1/2 teaspoon dried rosemary • Salt and pepper

Preparation Method: Baking

Directions:

- Bring your oven up to 375°F (190°C).
- Rub the chicken thigh with olive oil, rosemary, salt, and pepper.
- Bake for 30-35 minutes until cooked through.

Nutritional Values: • Calories: 250 • Fat: 12g (9g healthy fats, 3g unhealthy fats) • Carbohydrates: 0g • Fiber: 0g • Protein: 30g • Sugar: 0g

Recipe 2: Roasted Carrot and Parsnip Medley

Preparation Time: 30 minutes | **Servings**: 1

Ingredients: • 1/2 cup carrots, sliced • 1/2 cup parsnips, sliced • One teaspoon of olive oil • Half a teaspoon of dried thyme • Salt, to taste • Pepper, to taste

Preparation Method: Roasting

Directions:

- Bring your oven up to 400°F (200°C).
- Combine the vegetables with some oil, dried thyme, and a pinch of seasoning, ensuring they are evenly coated.
- Roast for 25-30 minutes until the vegetables are tender and caramelized.

Nutritional Values: • Calories: 130 • Fat: 4g (3g healthy fats, 1g unhealthy fats) • Carbohydrates: 20g • Fiber: 6g • Protein: 2g • Sugar: 7g

Recipe 3: Spinach and Feta Stuffed Bell Pepper

Preparation Time: 25 minutes | **Servings**: 1

Ingredients: • One small bell pepper halved • 1/4 cup cooked spinach • One tablespoon of crumbled feta cheese • One teaspoon of olive oil

Preparation Method: Baking

Directions:

- Bring the oven to 350°F (175°C).
- Stuff the bell pepper halves with cooked spinach and feta.
- Coat with oil and cook in the oven for 20-25 minutes until they achieve a golden-brown color.

Nutritional Values: • Calories: 140 • Fat: 8g (6g healthy fats, 2g unhealthy fats) • Carbohydrates: 10g • Fiber: 4g • Protein: 5g • Sugar: 5g

Recipe 4: Grilled Salmon Fillet

Preparation Time: 15 minutes | **Servings**: 1

Ingredients: • 1 salmon fillet (4 oz) • One teaspoon of olive oil • 1/2 teaspoon dried dill • Salt and pepper

Preparation Method: Grilling

Directions:

- Brush the salmon with olive oil, dill, salt, and pepper.
- Cook each side on medium heat for 5-7 minutes until perfectly grilled.

Nutritional Values: • Calories: 220 • Fat: 12g (10g healthy fats, 2g unhealthy fats) • Carbohydrates: 0g • Fiber: 0g • Protein: 24g • Sugar: 0g

Recipe 5: Sweet Potato and Apple Bake

Preparation Time: 30 minutes | **Servings:** 1

Ingredients: • 1/2 cup sweet potato, sliced • 1/2 apple, sliced • One teaspoon of olive oil • 1/2 teaspoon cinnamon

Preparation Method: Baking

Directions:

- Bring your oven up to 375°F (190°C).
- Toss the sweet potato and apple slices with olive oil and cinnamon.
- Cook for 25-30 minutes until the food is tender and caramelized.

Nutritional Values: • Calories: 140 • Fat: 4g (3g healthy fats, 1g unhealthy fats) • Carbohydrates: 28g • Fiber: 5g • Protein: 1g • Sugar: 10g

Conclusion

Special occasions are about more than just food—togetherness, celebration, and creating lasting memories. However, delicious meals often take center stage during these times, and it's essential to ensure that everyone, including those managing diabetes, can enjoy the feast without worry. The recipes in this chapter are crafted with care, offering flavorful, balanced, and healthy options that bring joy to the table while supporting blood sugar management.

From holiday spreads to family gatherings and casual entertaining, these diabetes-friendly recipes allow you to celebrate without compromising your health goals. Focusing on fresh, whole ingredients and thoughtful preparation ensures that these meals are both nourishing and satisfying for everyone.

Remember, special occasions are a time to celebrate the people in your life. Incorporating these recipes into your celebrations can create dishes that bring comfort and happiness while supporting well-being. Enjoying festive meals everyone can appreciate is possible with mindful choices and creativity.

Chapter 11: The 45-Day Meal Plan for Managing Type 2 Diabetes

Introduction

Embarking on the journey of managing Type 2 diabetes, particularly for those over 50, can be overwhelming. However, this 45-day meal plan is a guide and a tool designed to simplify your life, improve your health, and make your journey more enjoyable. It's more than just choosing what to eat; it's about making informed choices, stabilizing your blood sugar levels, and embracing a balanced lifestyle. This chapter equips you with essential tools—detailed shopping lists, daily schedules, and meal-prepping tips—to help you survive and thrive on this path. Meal planning promotes healthy eating habits, controls blood sugar levels, and simplifies daily food choices. This chapter provides everything you need, including weekly shopping lists, daily meal schedules, and practical meal-prepping tips. Let's get started on this journey to better health and wellbeing.

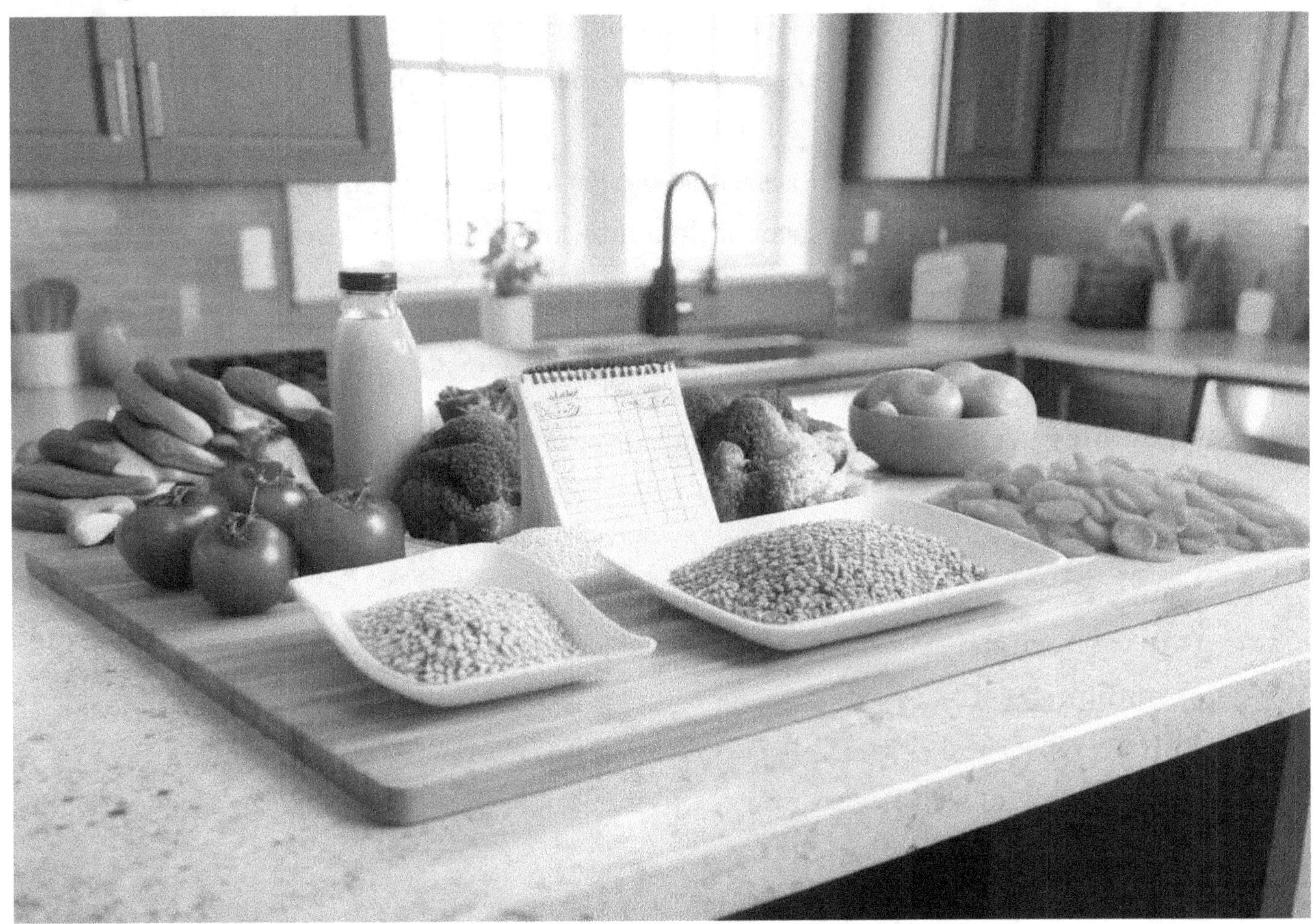

11.1: Weekly Shopping Lists

Our organized shopping lists ensure you possess all the vital ingredients to whip up nutritious meals throughout the week. These lists save you time and reduce the stress of last-minute grocery runs, helping you feel more organized and prepared. With everything planned out in advance, you can enjoy a smoother meal prep experience and focus on maintaining a healthy lifestyle.

Week 1 Shopping List

- **Fruits**: 7 apples, seven bananas, 1 pint of blueberries
- **Vegetables**: 1 lb Brussels sprouts, 1 lb green beans, one head cauliflower, three zucchinis, 2 lbs carrots
- **Proteins**: 3.3 lbs chicken breast, 1.1 lbs turkey meatballs, 12 eggs
- **Grains**: 1.1 lbs quinoa, 2.2 lbs brown rice
- **Dairy Alternatives**: 2.2 lbs Greek yogurt, 1-quart almond milk

Week 2 Shopping List

- **Fruits**: 2.2 lbs strawberries, seven kiwis, seven oranges
- **Vegetables**: 1.1 lbs bell peppers, 2.2 lbs tomatoes, 2.2 lbs spinach, 1.1 lbs broccoli, 2.2 lbs sweet potatoes
- **Proteins**: 2.2 lbs salmon, 1.1 lbs shrimp, 2.2 lbs lentils, 1.1 lbs chickpeas
- **Grains**: 1.1 lbs barley, 1.1 lbs coconut flour, one loaf whole grain bread
- **Dairy Alternatives**: 2.2 lbs coconut yogurt, 1.1 lbs almond butter

Week 3 Shopping List

- **Fruits**: 2.2 lbs grapes, one pineapple, six pears
- **Vegetables**: 1.1 lbs asparagus, 1.1 lbs mushrooms, one head of cabbage, four cucumbers, six avocados
- **Proteins**: 2.2 lbs cod, 1.1 lbs scallops, 1.1 lbs tofu
- **Grains**: 2.2 lbs brown rice, 2.2 lbs whole wheat pasta
- **Dairy Alternatives**: 1-quart soy milk, 1.1 kg vegan cheese

Week 4 Shopping List

- **Fruits**: 1.1 lbs blackberries, 1.1 lbs raspberries, two mangoes
- **Vegetables**: 1.1 lbs Brussels sprouts, 1.1 lbs green beans, 2.2 lbs carrots, three zucchinis, 1.1 lbs kale
- **Proteins**: 3.3 lbs chicken thighs, 1.1 lbs turkey sausages, 12 eggs

- **Grains**: 1.1 lbs quinoa, 2.2 lbs oats
- **Dairy Alternatives**: 2.2 lbs Greek yogurt, 1-quart coconut milk

<u>**Week 5 Shopping List**</u>

- **Fruits**: 7 apples, seven bananas, 1 pint of blueberries
- **Vegetables**: 1.1 lbs broccoli, 2.2 lbs spinach, one head cauliflower, 2.2 lbs tomatoes, 2.2 lbs sweet potatoes
- **Proteins**: 2.2 lbs beef, 2.2 lbs pork tenderloin, 2.2 lbs lentils
- **Grains**: 2.2 lbs brown rice, one loaf whole grain bread
- **Dairy Alternatives**: 1-quart almond milk, 2.2 kg dairy-free yogurt

<u>**Week 6 Shopping List**</u>

- **Fruits**: 7 oranges, seven kiwis, 2.2 lbs strawberries
- **Vegetables**: 1.1 lbs green peppers, 2.2 lbs onions, 2.2 lbs carrots, 1.1 lbs mushrooms, six avocados
- **Proteins**: 3.3 lbs chicken breast, 1.1 lbs tuna, 2.2 lbs chickpeas
- **Grains**: 1.1 lbs barley, one pack of whole wheat tortillas
- **Dairy Alternatives**: 2.2 lbs coconut yogurt, 1.1 lbs vegan cheese

<u>**Week 7 Shopping List**</u>

- **Fruits**: 1 small watermelon, 2.2 lbs grapes, one pineapple
- **Vegetables**: 2.2 lbs spinach, 1.1 lbs broccoli, 1.1 lbs kale, 2.2 lbs tomatoes, four cucumbers
- **Proteins**: 2.2 lbs salmon, 1.1 lbs shrimp, 12 eggs
- **Grains**: 1.1 lbs quinoa, 2.2 lbs brown rice
- **Dairy Alternatives**: 2.2 lbs Greek yogurt, 1.1 lbs almond butter

11.2: Daily Meal Schedules

Here's a detailed meal plan for the 45 days:

Day 1 Meal Schedule

- **Breakfast**: Veggie Omelet
- **Snack**: Greek Yogurt with Flaxseeds and Blueberries
- **Lunch**: Lentil Salad with Cucumber and Tomato
- **Snack**: Celery Sticks with Peanut Butter
- **Dinner**: Grilled Chicken Breast with Herbs

Day 2 Meal Schedule

- **Breakfast**: Peanut Butter and Banana Smoothie
- **Snack**: Hard-Boiled Eggs with Veggies
- **Lunch**: Tuna Salad with Avocado
- **Snack**: Almonds and Blueberries
- **Dinner**: Balsamic Glazed Roasted Brussels Sprouts

Day 3 Meal Schedule

- **Breakfast**: Scrambled Eggs with Smoked Salmon
- **Snack**: Apple and Cinnamon Compote
- **Lunch**: Quinoa Pilaf with Herbs
- **Snack**: Cucumber and Hummus Bites
- **Dinner**: Lentil and Spinach Stew

Day 4 Meal Schedule

- **Breakfast**: Avocado Cocoa Smoothie
- **Snack**: Greek Yogurt with Walnuts
- **Lunch**: Chickpea and Tomato Curry
- **Snack**: Cottage Cheese and Tomato Salad
- **Dinner**: Grilled Vegetable Quinoa Bowl

Day 5 Meal Schedule

- **Breakfast**: Cocoa Almond Smoothie
- **Snack**: Almond Butter Bites
- **Lunch**: Spinach and Chicken Salad
- **Snack**: Roasted Sweet Potato Wedges
- **Dinner**: Turkey Meatballs with Tomato Sauce

Day 6 Meal Schedule

- **Breakfast**: Tropical Smoothie
- **Snack**: Frozen Banana Bites
- **Lunch**: Greek Salad with Feta
- **Snack**: Hard-Boiled Eggs with Veggies
- **Dinner**: Beef Stir-Fry with Broccoli

Day 7 Meal Schedule

- **Breakfast**: Low-Carb Pancakes with Almond Flour
- **Snack**: Kiwi and Strawberry Salad

- **Lunch**: Baked Cod with Herbs
- **Snack**: Greek Yogurt with Flaxseeds and Blueberries
- **Dinner**: Pork Tenderloin with Garlic and Herbs

Day 8 Meal Schedule

- **Breakfast**: Spinach and Mushroom Scramble
- **Snack**: Cottage Cheese and Tomato Salad
- **Lunch**: Shrimp Stir-Fry with Vegetables
- **Snack**: Greek Yogurt with Walnuts
- **Dinner**: Baked Chicken Thigh with Lemon

Day 9 Meal Schedule

- **Breakfast**: Green Power Smoothie
- **Snack**: Celery Sticks with Peanut Butter
- **Lunch**: Barley with Mushrooms
- **Snack**: Almond Butter Bites
- **Dinner**: Roasted Carrots with Thyme

Day 10 Meal Schedule

- **Breakfast**: Sautéed Green Beans with Almonds
- **Snack**: Greek Yogurt with Flaxseeds and Blueberries
- **Lunch**: Brown Rice with Garlic and Spinach
- **Snack**: Hard-Boiled Eggs with Veggies
- **Dinner**: Chickpea and Red Pepper Stew

Day 11 Meal Schedule

- **Breakfast**: Lentil Salad with Cucumber and Tomato
- **Snack**: Greek Yogurt with Walnuts
- **Lunch**: Tomato and Lentil Soup
- **Snack**: Cottage Cheese and Tomato Salad
- **Dinner**: Pork Tenderloin with Garlic and Herbs

Day 12 Meal Schedule

- **Breakfast**: Scrambled Eggs with Smoked Salmon
- **Snack**: Greek Yogurt with Flaxseeds and Berries
- **Lunch**: Baked Eggplant Rounds with Parmesan
- **Snack**: Celery Sticks with Peanut Butter

- **Dinner**: Spinach and Chicken Salad

Day 13 Meal Schedule

- **Breakfast**: Peanut Butter and Banana Smoothie
- **Snack**: Greek Yogurt with Flaxseeds and Berries
- **Lunch**: Grilled Vegetable Quinoa Bowl
- **Snack**: Cucumber and Hummus Bites
- **Dinner**: Roasted Sweet Potato Wedges

Day 14 Meal Schedule

- **Breakfast**: Veggie Omelette
- **Snack**: Cottage Cheese and Tomato Salad
- **Lunch**: Tuna Salad with Avocado
- **Snack**: Almonds and Berries
- **Dinner**: Beef Stir-Fry with Broccoli

Day 15 Meal Schedule

- **Breakfast**: Berry Almond Smoothie
- **Snack**: Greek Yogurt with Flaxseeds and Berries
- **Lunch**: Baked Chicken Thigh with Lemon
- **Snack**: Celery Sticks with Peanut Butter
- **Dinner**: Grilled Salmon with Lemon

Day 16 Meal Schedule

- **Breakfast**: Tropical Smoothie
- **Snack**: Frozen Banana Bites
- **Lunch**: Greek Salad with Feta
- **Snack**: Hard-boiled Eggs with Veggies
- **Dinner**: Seared Scallops with Asparagus

Day 17 Meal Schedule

- **Breakfast**: Cocoa Almond Smoothie
- **Snack**: Almond Butter Bites
- **Lunch**: Chickpea and Tomato Curry
- **Snack**: Cottage Cheese and Tomato Salad
- **Dinner**: Grilled Zucchini with Parmesan

Day 18 Meal Schedule

- **Breakfast**: Scrambled Eggs with Smoked Salmon

- **Snack**: Greek Yogurt with Flaxseeds and Berries
- **Lunch**: Turkey Meatballs with Tomato Sauce
- **Snack**: Cucumber and Hummus Bites
- **Dinner**: Tuna and Avocado Sandwich

Day 19 Meal Schedule

- **Breakfast**: Avocado and Egg Toast
- **Snack**: Cottage Cheese and Tomato Salad
- **Lunch**: Brown Rice with Garlic and Spinach
- **Snack**: Greek Yogurt with Walnuts
- **Dinner**: Roasted Sweet Potato Wedges

Day 20 Meal Schedule

- **Breakfast**: Peanut Butter and Banana Smoothie
- **Snack**: Hard-Boiled Eggs with Veggies
- **Lunch**: Chickpea and Red Pepper Stew
- **Snack**: Almonds and Berries
- **Dinner**: Shrimp Stir-Fry with Vegetables

Day 21 Meal Schedule

- **Breakfast**: Green Power Smoothie
- **Snack**: Celery Sticks with Peanut Butter
- **Lunch**: Quinoa Pilaf with Herbs
- **Snack**: Greek Yogurt with Walnuts
- **Dinner**: Turkey and Avocado Wrap

Day 22 Meal Schedule

- **Breakfast**: Low-Carb Pancakes with Almond Flour
- **Snack**: Kiwi and Strawberry Salad
- **Lunch**: Baked Cod with Herbs
- **Snack**: Greek Yogurt with Flaxseeds and Berries
- **Dinner**: Pork Tenderloin with Garlic and Herbs

Day 23 Meal Schedule

- **Breakfast**: Veggie Omelette
- **Snack**: Greek Yogurt with Flaxseeds and Berries
- **Lunch**: Tomato and Lentil Soup

- **Snack**: Cottage Cheese and Tomato Salad
- **Dinner**: Beef Stir-Fry with Broccoli

Day 24 Meal Schedule

- **Breakfast**: Scrambled Eggs with Smoked Salmon
- **Snack**: Greek Yogurt with Flaxseeds and Berries
- **Lunch**: Baked Eggplant Rounds with Parmesan
- **Snack**: Celery Sticks with Peanut Butter
- **Dinner**: Spinach and Chicken Salad

Day 25 Meal Schedule

- **Breakfast**: Cocoa Almond Smoothie
- **Snack**: Almond Butter Bites
- **Lunch**: Tuna Salad with Avocado
- **Snack**: Hard-Boiled Eggs with Veggies
- **Dinner**: Grilled Zucchini with Parmesan

Day 26 Meal Schedule

- **Breakfast**: Tropical Smoothie
- **Snack**: Frozen Banana Bites
- **Lunch**: Greek Salad with Feta
- **Snack**: Hard-boiled Eggs with Veggies
- **Dinner**: Seared Scallops with Asparagus

Day 27 Meal Schedule

- **Breakfast**: Peanut Butter and Banana Smoothie
- **Snack**: Greek Yogurt with Flaxseeds and Berries
- **Lunch**: Turkey Meatballs with Tomato Sauce
- **Snack**: Almonds and Berries
- **Dinner**: Chickpea and Tomato Curry

Day 28 Meal Schedule

- **Breakfast**: Avocado Cocoa Smoothie
- **Snack**: Greek Yogurt with Walnuts
- **Lunch**: Grilled Vegetable Quinoa Bowl
- **Snack**: Cottage Cheese and Tomato Salad
- **Dinner**: Baked Cod with Herbs

Day 29 Meal Schedule

- **Breakfast**: Green Power Smoothie
- **Snack**: Celery Sticks with Peanut Butter
- **Lunch**: Brown Rice with Garlic and Spinach
- **Snack**: Greek Yogurt with Walnuts
- **Dinner**: Beef Stir-Fry with Broccoli

Day 30 Meal Schedule

- **Breakfast**: Low-Carb Pancakes with Almond Flour
- **Snack**: Kiwi and Strawberry Salad
- **Lunch**: Tomato and Lentil Soup
- **Snack**: Cottage Cheese and Tomato Salad
- **Dinner**: Grilled Chicken Breast with Herbs

Day 31 Meal Schedule

- **Breakfast**: Veggie Omelette
- **Snack**: Greek Yogurt with Flaxseeds and Berries
- **Lunch**: Tuna Salad with Avocado
- **Snack**: Almonds and Berries
- **Dinner**: Shrimp Stir-Fry with Vegetables

Day 32 Meal Schedule

- **Breakfast**: Peanut Butter and Banana Smoothie
- **Snack**: Hard-Boiled Eggs with Veggies
- **Lunch**: Lentil Salad with Cucumber and Tomato
- **Snack**: Celery Sticks with Peanut Butter
- **Dinner**: Balsamic Glazed Roasted Brussels Sprouts

Day 33 Meal Schedule

- **Breakfast**: Scrambled Eggs with Smoked Salmon
- **Snack**: Greek Yogurt with Flaxseeds and Berries
- **Lunch**: Quinoa Pilaf with Herbs
- **Snack**: Cucumber and Hummus Bites
- **Dinner**: Lentil and Spinach Stew

Day 34 Meal Schedule

- **Breakfast**: Avocado Cocoa Smoothie
- **Snack**: Greek Yogurt with Walnuts

- **Lunch**: Chickpea and Tomato Curry
- **Snack**: Cottage Cheese and Tomato Salad
- **Dinner**: Grilled Vegetable Quinoa Bowl

Day 35 Meal Schedule

- **Breakfast**: Cocoa Almond Smoothie
- **Snack**: Almond Butter Bites
- **Lunch**: Spinach and Chicken Salad
- **Snack**: Roasted Sweet Potato Wedges
- **Dinner**: Turkey Meatballs with Tomato Sauce

Day 36 Meal Schedule

- **Breakfast**: Tropical Smoothie
- **Snack**: Frozen Banana Bites
- **Lunch**: Greek Salad with Feta
- **Snack**: Hard-boiled Eggs with Veggies
- **Dinner**: Beef Stir-Fry with Broccoli

Day 37 Meal Schedule

- **Breakfast**: Low-Carb Pancakes with Almond Flour
- **Snack**: Kiwi and Strawberry Salad
- **Lunch**: Baked Cod with Herbs
- **Snack**: Greek Yogurt with Flaxseeds and Berries
- **Dinner**: Pork Tenderloin with Garlic and Herbs

Day 38 Meal Schedule

- **Breakfast**: Green Power Smoothie
- **Snack**: Celery Sticks with Peanut Butter
- **Lunch**: Barley with Mushrooms
- **Snack**: Greek Yogurt with Walnuts
- **Dinner**: Roasted Carrots with Thyme

Day 39 Meal Schedule

- **Breakfast**: Scrambled Eggs with Smoked Salmon
- **Snack**: Greek Yogurt with Flaxseeds and Berries
- **Lunch**: Brown Rice with Garlic and Spinach
- **Snack**: Cottage Cheese and Tomato Salad
- **Dinner**: Chickpea and Red Pepper Stew

Day 40 Meal Schedule

- **Breakfast**: Berry Almond Smoothie
- **Snack**: Greek Yogurt with Flaxseeds and Berries
- **Lunch**: Baked Chicken Thigh with Lemon
- **Snack**: Celery Sticks with Peanut Butter
- **Dinner**: Grilled Salmon with Lemon

Day 41 Meal Schedule

- **Breakfast**: Tropical Smoothie
- **Snack**: Frozen Banana Bites
- **Lunch**: Greek Salad with Feta
- **Snack**: Hard-boiled Eggs with Veggies
- **Dinner**: Seared Scallops with Asparagus

Day 42 Meal Schedule

- **Breakfast**: Cocoa Almond Smoothie
- **Snack**: Almond Butter Bites
- **Lunch**: Chickpea and Tomato Curry
- **Snack**: Cottage Cheese and Tomato Salad
- **Dinner**: Grilled Zucchini with Parmesan

Day 43 Meal Schedule

- **Breakfast**: Scrambled Eggs with Smoked Salmon
- **Snack**: Greek Yogurt with Flaxseeds and Berries
- **Lunch**: Turkey Meatballs with Tomato Sauce
- **Snack**: Cucumber and Hummus Bites
- **Dinner**: Tuna and Avocado Sandwich

Day 44 Meal Schedule

- **Breakfast**: Avocado and Egg Toast
- **Snack**: Cottage Cheese and Tomato Salad
- **Lunch**: Brown Rice with Garlic and Spinach
- **Snack**: Greek Yogurt with Walnuts
- **Dinner**: Grilled Chicken Breast with Herbs

Day 45 Meal Schedule

- **Breakfast**: Green Power Smoothie

- **Snack**: Celery Sticks with Peanut Butter
- **Lunch**: Barley with Mushrooms
- **Snack**: Almond Butter Bites
- **Dinner**: Roasted Carrots with Thyme

11.3: Tips for Meal Prepping

Efficient meal preparation can save time, reduce stress, and promote healthier eating habits.

Plan your weekly menu: Dedicate a day to planning your meals and another day to cooking.

Use clear containers: Store prepped meals and snacks in see-through containers to quickly find what you need.

Label meals with dates: Monitor the freshness of your food to prevent waste.

Batch cooking: Prepare large quantities of staples like grains, beans, and proteins, then portion them out for the week.

Make use of leftovers: Incorporate leftovers into new meals to be more efficient and reduce waste.

Conclusion

Completing a structured **45-day meal plan** manages Type 2 diabetes while enjoying nutritious and delicious meals. By following this plan, you've taken a proactive step towards balancing blood sugar levels, promoting overall health, and simplifying your daily food choices. The provided meals and snacks combine diverse flavors, textures, and essential nutrients, all carefully crafted to meet your dietary needs.

Each week of this plan introduces a combination of proteins, healthy fats, fiber-rich carbohydrates, and fresh fruits and vegetables, ensuring your diet remains balanced and enjoyable. Whether cooking for yourself or enjoying meals with loved ones, these recipes are crafted to be simple to prepare and customizable to fit your tastes.

The weekly **shopping lists** provide a practical way to organize your groceries, ensuring you have all the necessary ingredients to prepare each meal without stress. From hearty breakfasts and satisfying lunches to flavorful dinners and energizing snacks, this meal plan covers every aspect of your day-to-day eating.

You can rotate recipes, explore new flavors, and find the best combinations. By sticking to a thoughtful and well-organized meal plan, you'll continue to enjoy both the short-term and long-term benefits of managing your diabetes through smart, delicious choices. As you move forward, feel empowered to maintain this routine and make healthy eating a regular part of your life.

You've proven that with the right approach, managing diabetes can be a positive, satisfying experience that keeps you energized, nourished, and feeling your best.

Chapter 12: Implementing Changes and Overcoming Challenges

Introduction

Adjusting to a new eating routine, particularly for managing Type 2 diabetes, can feel overwhelming. For those over 50, adapting to healthier habits often involves unlearning decades of old routines and adopting new, more mindful approaches to food. This process requires change, patience, determination, and willingness to embrace these changes.

This chapter will discuss the practical steps to transition into a diabetes-friendly diet and overcome common hurdles smoothly. From adjusting to new eating habits and managing social and family meals to staying motivated throughout the journey, you'll find realistic and empowering strategies. The key is approaching each change as an opportunity to build healthier, more sustainable habits that will ultimately support your long-term well-being. Remember, making these adjustments isn't about perfection but about progress. Every small change you make matters, and this section will provide you with practical tips and supportive insights to empower you on your journey to better health.

12.1: Adjusting to New Eating Habits

Adjusting to a new way of eating doesn't have to happen simultaneously. Gradually making thoughtful changes can ease the transition and make it more sustainable in the long run. Here are some practical tips to guide you toward a diabetes-friendly diet without feeling overwhelmed:

Start Small

Rather than overhauling your entire diet overnight, focus on replacing unhealthy habits one step at a time. Start by swapping out high-sugar snacks for healthier options like nuts, fruits, or yogurt. Remember, every small change you make counts, and this way, you can build better habits that will gradually take root, empowering you to manage your health.

Incorporate More Vegetables

Aim to add more vegetables to your meals. Try making half your plate vegetables at lunch and dinner. Over time, this minor adjustment can significantly improve your overall nutrient intake while helping regulate blood sugar levels.

Experiment with New Recipes

Getting creative in the kitchen can make transitioning to healthier eating more enjoyable. Explore new recipes, spices, and cooking methods that support your dietary objectives. Don't hesitate to make substitutions in your favorite recipes—whole grains instead of refined grains, baked instead of fried. These minor adjustments can lead to noticeable improvements.

Focus on Balance

Ensure your meals are balanced with carbs, proteins, and beneficial fats to keep your blood glucose stable. Consider meals that combine quinoa or brown rice as whole grains, chicken or tofu for lean proteins, and avocado or nuts for healthy fats. This balanced approach ensures you get the essential nutrients and supports stable glucose levels.

12.2: Dealing with Social and Family Meals

When sticking to a new dietary plan, social gatherings and family meals can present challenges. Whether it's holidays, birthdays, or simply dinner with friends, these situations often involve food that may not align with your diabetes management goals. Here are some strategies to help you navigate these occasions while still enjoying yourself:

Bring a Diabetes-Friendly Dish

When attending a potluck or family meal, bringing a dish you know is safe to eat ensures you have at least one option that meets your dietary needs. Plus, it allows you to introduce others to tasty, healthy alternatives they might not have tried before.

Communicate Your Needs

Communicating openly with family and friends about your dietary preferences is essential. You don't have to explain every detail, but letting others know about your health goals can encourage them to offer support or make accommodationsIf you feel pressured to eat something that doesn't align with your goals, you can politely decline and explain that you're focusing on healthier eating to manage your diabetes. Most people will respect your decision.

Practice Portion Control

Celebrations often include tempting foods that are hard to ignore. Instead of avoiding these indulgences altogether, try practicing portion control. You can enjoy small servings of your favorite dishes without feeling deprived. Pair them with a healthy salad or vegetable to maintain healthy habits.

Stay Mindful of Hidden Sugars

Be mindful of hidden sugars lurking in condiments, sauces, and dressings at gatherings. Opt for simple, fresh foods where possible; if unsure about the ingredients, it's okay to ask. This reassurance lets you make confident and informed choices about your meals, giving you control over your dietary preferences.

12.3: Keeping Motivated

Maintaining motivation is often the most challenging part of making long-term changes. When managing diabetes, it's crucial to stay committed even when the journey gets tough. Here are a few ways to keep your motivation strong and your mindset positive:

Set Realistic Goals

Break your overall health goals into bite-sized, achievable steps. For example, rather than aiming to 'completely change your diet,' start with a specific goal like 'incorporate more vegetables into my meals' or 'limit added sugars.'

Don't be too hard on yourself if you have a setback or lapse in your diet. It's normal to have occasional slip-ups. Instead, use it as a learning experience and a chance to recommit to your goals. Once you achieve one small goal, you'll feel more confident moving on to the next.

Track Your Progress

Recording your meals or using an app to monitor them can make a big difference. It helps you keep track of your dietary choices, see what's working, where adjustments might be needed, and understand how different foods make you feel. Tracking your physical and emotional progress can serve as a significant motivator.

Celebrate Small Wins

Recognize and celebrate each milestone, regardless of its size. Whether it's a successful week of balanced meals or discovering a new favorite healthy recipe, rewarding yourself for positive choices can boost your motivation. These small celebrations can reinforce your commitment to long-term success.

Build a Support System

Having support from family, friends, or a dedicated diabetes community can significantly contribute to your success. Surround yourself with people who encourage you and share your journey. This sense of community and shared experience creates a support system, keeping you accountable and inspired, making you feel less alone and more connected.

Conclusion

Recap of Key Points

To wrap up our journey through Diabetic Diet After 50, let's focus on the essential insights to help manage Type 2 diabetes and boost overall well-being. The most vital takeaway is that diet is central to controlling blood diet levels and maintaining long-term health. For individuals over 50, this means paying close attention to nutritional needs that evolve with age and making conscious, informed food choices. From learning about the effects of carbohydrates, proteins, and fats on blood sugar to mastering meal planning and portion control, you now have practical strategies to manage your condition effectively. By embracing the principles of a diabetes-friendly diet, you're not only managing your diabetes but also supporting your body in achieving a better quality of life. By focusing on balanced nutrition, planning, and maintaining a positive mindset, you can take charge of your health and savor the foods you love. This approach aligns with your long-term goals and promotes overall well-being.

Continuing Your Journey

Managing diabetes is a lifelong journey; while there may be challenges, your progress is worth every effort. Remember, it's not about perfection—taking small, consistent steps that gradually lead to significant improvements. As you continue to integrate these dietary changes, stay flexible, be patient with yourself, and celebrate your achievements, no matter how small they may seem.

Challenges are a natural part of the process, but so is your ability to adapt and grow stronger. You have the strength within you to overcome these challenges. Set new goals as you move forward, and seek the support you need to stay motivated—whether from family, friends, or a diabetes community. Remember that each healthy choice you make contributes to a healthier future. This journey is about embracing positive change; you have all the tools to succeed.

Additional Resources

Your journey toward better health doesn't end here. There's always more to explore, including managing diabetes and living a balanced life. Consider diving deeper into topics related to diabetic-friendly nutrition, meal planning, and holistic health. Books like 'The Diabetic Cookbook' and websites like 'Diabetes.org' offer valuable insights, but don't underestimate the power of communication. Participating in local diabetes groups or online forums like 'Diabetes Daily' can effectively share your experiences, get answers to your questions, and receive support from others facing similar challenges. Additionally, staying informed by attending community health events or participating in educational seminars can keep you engaged and motivated. The more you learn about diabetes management, the more prepared you'll be to make long-term decisions that enhance your health and well-being.

With the knowledge and strategies from this book, you're not just equipped but empowered to continue your journey toward better health. Embrace each day with the confidence that comes from understanding your body and making choices that support your health. You've already taken the first step—keep moving forward!

Acknowledgments

I want to take a moment to thank you for choosing **"DIABETIC DIET AFTER 50"** and for trusting this book to guide you on your journey toward better health. Writing this book has been a rewarding experience, and I hope the insights, recipes, and strategies within these pages help you feel empowered and confident in managing your diabetes. Your dedication to making healthier choices and enhancing your well-being is inspiring. Remember, you are the key player in your health journey. I extend my heartfelt gratitude to all who have shared their stories, challenges, and triumphs in managing diabetes. I also want to acknowledge the health professionals, nutritionists, and diabetes educators who continue to work tirelessly to improve the lives of people with this condition. Your knowledge and commitment have shaped the information, and I'm deeply grateful.

Finally, I'd love to hear your feedback! If this book has benefited you, leaving a review would be greatly appreciated. Your thoughts and insights can help others discover the value of this guide and encourage them to take control of their health. I appreciate your participation in this journey—your health is worth every step!